# Real-World Evidence: Principles and Practice

# Real-World Evidence: Principles and Practice

A Comprehensive Guide to the Science, Strategy, and Application of Real-World Evidence for Healthcare, Pharma, Regulatory, and HTA Professionals

**Massoud Toussi, MD, PhD, MBA**

**Real-World Evidence: Principles and Practice**



Elixir Institute

ISBN: 979-8-9948235-0-7

# Book Reviews

*"Massoud Toussi shares his immense experience in applying RWE to a wide range of relevant use cases. Anybody new to the field, whether HTA, regulatory, industry, or research, will benefit from a read."*

***Sebastian Schneeweiss, Chief, Division of Pharmacoepidemiology and Pharmacoeconomics, Harvard***

*"This book is a beautifully organized and easy-to-digest overview of RWE and its interplay with the complex world we navigate. It brings great clarity to this evolving field, helps join the dots, and shines light on where we need to focus now and what's coming next."*

***Noah Jamie Robinson, Executive Director, Head of Epidemiology & PV, Astellas***

*"Finally, a book that takes a holistic approach to the role of RWE throughout the entire product lifecycle. From market access to pricing and post-market surveillance - the practical examples and strategic insights are invaluable for anyone working in Life Sciences today. If you want to understand how real-world data is transforming our industry, start here."*

***Mats Rosenlund, Vice President, Global HEOR & RWE, Daiichi Saynkyo***

*"A comprehensive review of all types of real-world data sources, methodological aspects and practical considerations for implementation of RWE. Dr Toussi delivers a useful toolkit for researchers from industry and academia who are interested to explore standards and innovative methods."*

***Stéphanie Tcherny-Lessenot, Global Head of Epidemiology and Benefit-Risk ad Interim, Sanofi***

*"A comprehensive primer that summarizes the rapidly evolving state-of-the-art for rigorous investigation of real-word data sources to inform decision-making by clinicians, researchers, payers, regulatory and HTA authorities. This is a valuable resource for both experienced decision-makers and students alike."*

**Marc Berger, Vice President Emeritus, Real World Data and Analytics, Pfizer**

*"RWE has the potential to radically accelerate the way we operate, providing stakeholders align on expectations. Massoud Toussi brings a unique RWE one-stop-shop (data sources, methodologies, assessment) which could do just that."*

**Dana Vigier, President & General Manager, France, Belgium & Luxembourg, Alexion Pharmaceuticals**

*"This book is a compendium of all aspects of RWE generation, from study concept to strategic applications. I highly recommend it as a source for all players in the field where RWE is applied, including regulatory, payer, and health technology bodies."*

**Ayad Ali, Head of Global Safety Epidemiology, BeOne Medicines**

*"A useful guide to understanding pharmacoepidemiology and its applications for studying effectiveness, safety and value."*

**Nancy Dreyer, Chief Scientific Officer Emerita, IQVIA Real-World Solutions**

## START THE JOURNEY

This book is more than a standalone volume—it is an invitation into a living learning ecosystem. At **Evidence Mastery™**, the journey starts: deepen your expertise with companion titles, masterclasses, and actionable templates; stay inspired through our **LinkedIn newsletter** and **YouTube channel**; and accelerate your work with curated guidelines, databases, and AI-powered tools via **EvidenceAi™ Suite**. Every resource is designed to transform insight into impact—because evidence, when elevated by community and technology, becomes a catalyst for change. Welcome to the next level of mastery.

Scan to explore evidencemastery.com

# Table of Contents

# Preface

Less than two decades ago, "real-world evidence" was a phrase whispered in conference corridors - a promising but peripheral concept. Today, it anchors regulatory approvals, shapes value-based contracts, and guides public health policy worldwide. The journey from niche curiosity to embedded practice has been extraordinary, and I have had the privilege of witnessing - and contributing to - this transformation from its earliest days.

Real-world evidence has now matured into a discipline of its own. Yet practitioners are still expected to assemble its foundations - drawing from epidemiology, biostatistics, health economics, HEOR, market access, regulatory science and data science - only to find that critical integration gaps remain. Too many clinicians, medical affairs teams, HTA analysts, and students navigate by intuition, precedent, or fragmented guidelines. They face recurring, high-stakes questions: *Which study design is truly fit-for-purpose? How do I align evidence generation with stakeholder decision criteria? What makes RWE credible - not just statistically sound, but strategically relevant?*

This book was written to answer those questions. Not as a catalogue of methods, but as a coherent practice guide. Its central premise is that RWE must be purpose-built: anchored in stakeholder needs, disciplined by lifecycle context, and validated by fitness-for-use. The structure reflects this philosophy. We begin with foundations - What is RWE? Where is it used? Who are the stakeholders? - before examining study designs, bias control, and critical appraisal. Later chapters explore practical domains - regulatory, health technology assessment, clinical, pharmaceutical, evidence strategy planning - and emerging frontiers: digital health, AI, and continuous evidence generation. Throughout, examples from the U.S., Europe, Japan, and low-resource settings illustrate how theory translates into practice.

A single volume cannot capture a living discipline. To support continuous methodological development, this book is accompanied by a structured scholarly ecosystem at evidencemastery.com: updated case studies, template libraries, methodological guidelines, and tools designed to bridge theory and practice. These resources exist to organize a field that has expanded faster than its training infrastructure, and to equip practitioners with reproducible, decision-ready frameworks.

This book is not a replacement for regulatory guidance, statistical textbooks, or epidemiology primers. It is a translator: rendering complex principles into actionable insights, distinguishing signal from noise, and empowering you to design, evaluate, and apply RWE with confidence. Despite rigorous efforts to ensure accuracy - including verification of references, data sources, case examples and regulatory guidelines - this work may contain inadvertent errors or evolving discrepancies, given the pace of methodological and regulatory change. I welcome scholarly dialogue and constructive feedback. Readers who identify methodological updates, regulatory shifts, or opportunities for refinement are encouraged to share observations via professional correspondence or direct messaging. Contributions will inform future editions and strengthen collective practice.

On a personal note, writing this book has been a journey of conviction and compromise. I am deeply grateful to the many collaborators, regulators, clinicians, and patients who have shaped my understanding of this field over years of shared work. I also extend my sincere thanks to the friends and colleagues who generously reviewed early drafts - their thoughtful critiques, encouraging words, and sharp attention to detail elevated this work in countless ways. You know who you are, and I am honored by your support.

My family has been my quiet foundation throughout this process. To my wife, Virginie, whose patience and wisdom steadied me through countless late nights. To my sons, Daniel and Benjamin, who accepted my absences with grace and reminded me daily why evidence matters: for the world they will inherit. I also thank my mother, whose stay during the final drafting months with us provided both grounding and gentle reminders that life continues beyond the page. Many weekends, she and the family stepped out while I remained with citations and revisions. Their quiet support made this possible. And to my father, who first believed I had something to say. When I was nineteen, he encouraged me to publish my first book, teaching me early on that curiosity, discipline, and intellectual courage are the foundations of any worthwhile endeavor. I still miss him, and his belief in rigorous, transparent knowledge continues to guide me.

The journey from data to decision is rarely linear. But with principled practice, it can be trustworthy. And with community, it can be transformative.

Welcome to the next level of mastery.

*Massoud Toussi*

May 2026

# Part I: Foundations of Real-World Evidence

# Chapter 1. What Is Real-World Evidence?

In the evolving landscape of healthcare decision-making, a paradigm shift is underway - from reliance on highly controlled experimental data to the strategic integration of information generated during routine clinical practice. This shift is embodied in the concept of **Real-World Evidence (RWE)**. At its core, RWE represents the clinical evidence regarding the usage, benefits, and risks of medical products derived from the analysis of **Real-World Data (RWD)**. But what precisely constitutes RWD, and how does it transform into meaningful evidence?

The U.S. Food and Drug Administration (FDA) provides a widely adopted working definition:

*"Real-world data (RWD) are data relating to patient health status and/or the delivery of health care routinely collected from a variety of sources. Real-world evidence (RWE) is the clinical evidence about the usage and potential benefits or risks of a medical product derived from analysis of RWD"* [1].

The European Medicines Agency (EMA) provides a similar definition:

*"Real-World Data (RWD) are routinely collected data relating to patient health status or the delivery of health care from a variety of sources other than traditional clinical trials (e.g. claims databases, hospital data, electronic health records, registries, M-health data, etc.). Real-World Evidence is evidence derived from the analysis of RWD"* [2].

These definitions converge on some key elements:

- **Routine collection:** RWD are not generated for a clinical trial.
- **Diverse sources:** RWD can originate from observational studies, electronic health records (EHRs), claims and billing data, product and disease registries, patient-generated data (including from wearables and mobile health apps), and even social determinants of health databases.
- **Analytical transformation:** Raw data is not evidence. It becomes evidence afterwards.

The **scope of RWE** spans the entire product lifecycle - from pre-market development to product maturity and loss of patent.

It can inform:

- Regulatory decisions (e.g., label expansions, post-marketing requirements)
- Coverage and reimbursement policies by payers
- Clinical practice guidelines
- Public health surveillance
- Patient-centered care and shared decision-making
- Business related questions of the product owner

Critically, RWD is not synonymous with "observational data." While observational studies are a common source, RWD also includes data from electronic health records (EHRs), claims data, pragmatic clinical trials (PCTs) - studies that blend elements of RCTs with real-world settings - and increasingly, from digital biomarkers and wearables. The International Society for Pharmacoeconomics and Outcomes

Research (ISPOR) emphasizes that RWE must be **fit-for-purpose**, meaning the data and methods must align with the specific regulatory, clinical, or policy question at hand.

As healthcare systems globally grapple with rising costs, aging populations, and the need for personalized medicine, the demand for evidence that reflects actual patient experiences - across diverse demographics, comorbidities, and care settings - has never been greater. RWE fills this gap by capturing the complexity of real-life clinical practice, where treatment adherence is imperfect, polypharmacy is common, and outcomes are influenced by socioeconomic and environmental factors rarely accounted for in traditional trials.

## 1.1. RWE vs. RCTs: Complementary, Not Competitive

For decades, the **Randomized Controlled Trial (RCT)** has stood as the gold standard for establishing causal relationships between interventions and outcomes. RCTs achieve internal validity through randomization, blinding, strict inclusion/exclusion criteria, and protocol-driven interventions. These features minimize bias and confounding, making RCTs exceptionally powerful for demonstrating **efficacy** - that is, whether an intervention works under ideal conditions.

However, the very strengths of RCTs can limit their **external validity** or **generalizability**. Trial participants are often highly selected (e.g., excluding elderly patients, those with multiple comorbidities, or from underrepresented racial/ethnic groups), interventions are administered with perfect adherence, and outcomes are measured over short timeframes in specialized centers. Consequently, RCT findings may not reflect how a drug or device performs in routine practice - its **effectiveness**.

This is where RWE steps in. As summarized in Table 1.1 Key differences between RCT and RWE, RWE and RCTs serve distinct but complementary roles:

Rather than positioning RWE as a "lesser" alternative to RCTs, modern regulatory science embraces a **continuum of evidence**.

Regulators increasingly advocate for an integrated approach: RCTs establish initial safety and efficacy, while RWE extends understanding to broader populations, long-term outcomes, rare adverse events, and comparative effectiveness.

**Table 1.1 Key differences between RCT and RWE**

| Feature | Randomized Controlled Trials (RCTs) | Real-World Evidence (RWE) |
|---|---|---|
| **Primary goal** | Establish efficacy and safety under ideal conditions | Assess epidemiology, effectiveness, safety, use, acceptance in routine care |
| **Study population** | Homogeneous, narrowly defined | Heterogeneous, representative of real patients |
| **Intervention** | Standardized, protocol-driven | Variable, as prescribed in practice |
| **Setting** | Controlled, academic or trial centers | Diverse: clinics, hospitals, community, home |
| **Data collection** | Prospective, structured, high fidelity | Retrospective/prospective, unstructured/hybrid |
| **Time horizon** | Typically short-term | Can be long-term (chronic disease monitoring) |
| **Bias control** | Randomization, blinding | Statistical scoring, weighting and adjustment, advanced methods |
| **Regulatory role** | Primary basis for initial approval | Supports labeling, safety, coverage and commercial decisions |

Notably, the line between RCTs and RWE is blurred through **pragmatic clinical trials (PCTs)**. PCTs retain randomization but are embedded in real-world settings, use broad eligibility criteria, and measure patient-centered outcomes [3]. The NIH Health Care Systems Research Collaboratory has developed extensive guidance through real example, for conducting PCTs, emphasizing feasibility, stakeholder engagement, and minimal disruption to care [4].

Moreover, RWE can **inform** RCT design - by identifying relevant patient subgroups, selecting meaningful endpoints, or estimating event rates for sample size calculations. Conversely, RCT data can be used to validate RWE methodologies, ensuring that observational findings approximate causal truths.

The critical distinction lies not in data "quality" per se, but in **fitness for purpose**. An RCT is unfit to answer, "*How does this drug affect hospitalization rates in frail elderly patients with five comorbidities?*" just as an unadjusted claims database analysis is unfit to prove causality for a novel mechanism of action. *The method must match the question.*

## 1.2. Why RWE Matters in Modern Healthcare

The imperative for RWE arises from fundamental shifts in healthcare delivery, regulation, and patient expectations. Five converging forces make RWE not just useful, but essential:

1. **The Complexity of Modern Patients and Treatments**

   Today's patients are older, with multiple chronic conditions, and often take numerous medications. Monotherapy trials in young, healthy volunteers cannot predict outcomes in this reality. RWE captures polypharmacy interactions, treatment sequences, and real-world adherence patterns - critical for safe and effective prescribing.

2. **The Need for Long-Term and Rare Event Safety Data**

   Many serious adverse events (e.g., cardiovascular risks, rare cancers) emerge only after thousands of patient-years of exposure. RCTs, typically lasting months to a few years, are underpowered to detect such signals. Post-marketing surveillance using RWE - such as the FDA's Sentinel Initiative [5] - enables near real-time safety monitoring across millions of patients.

3. **Value-Based Healthcare and Payer Decisions**

   Payers (e.g., private insurers, national health services) demand evidence of **value**: *does a therapy improve outcomes relative to its cost in actual practice*? RWE informs health technology assessments (HTAs) by providing data on comparative effectiveness, quality of life, and resource utilization. The International Society for Pharmacoeconomics and Outcomes Research (ISPOR) has published extensive guidance on using RWE in HTA submissions [6, 7].

4. **Patient-Centered Outcomes and Shared Decision-Making**

   Patients increasingly seek information beyond "*Does it work?*" to "*Will it work for someone like me?*" RWE, especially from patient registries and digital health tools, captures patient-reported outcomes (PROs), functional status, and treatment burden - key inputs for personalized care plans.

5. **Accelerating Innovation and Regulatory Flexibility**

   Regulators are increasingly accepting RWE to support regulatory decisions. The 21st Century Cures Act (2016) mandated the FDA to evaluate RWE for potential use in labeling expansions [8]. The landmark example is the 2021 expansion of indication of tacrolimus to include organ rejection in patients receiving lung transplants, based solely on RWE generated from a patient registry [9].

The EMA and health technology bodies like NICE (UK) and CADTH (Canada) have similarly developed frameworks for RWE use [2,10]. This regulatory openness reflects a recognition that timely access to effective therapies should not be delayed by the limitations of traditional trial paradigms - provided the evidence is robust.

## 1.3. Evidence Pluralism: Embracing a Broader Epistemology

The rise of RWE is part of a larger philosophical movement in evidence-based medicine: **evidence pluralism**. Historically, hierarchies of evidence (e.g., GRADE, Oxford CEBM) placed RCTs and meta-analyses at the pinnacle, often dismissing observational studies as inherently biased. While this hierarchy protects against false positives in efficacy claims, it risks ignoring valuable insights about real-world performance, equity, and implementation.

Evidence pluralism or using the "totality of evidence" challenges this monolithic view. It posits that *different types of evidence answer different types of questions*, and that robust decision-making requires integrating multiple sources [11]. For instance:

- **Causal questions** (e.g., "*Does Drug X reduce stroke risk?*") may require RCTs with or without external RWE arms, or carefully designed RWE studies with strong causal inference methods.
- **Descriptive questions** (e.g., "*How is Drug X used in rural clinics?*") are best answered by RWD analytics i.e. raw data with basic analyses.
- **Implementation questions** (e.g., "*What barriers prevent uptake of a new guideline?*") demand qualitative and mixed-methods RWE.

This pluralistic approach is reflected in modern guidelines and emphasizes that study design should be driven by the research question, not preconceived notions of evidence "rank.". Similarly, the **RECORD Statement** (Reporting of Studies Conducted Using Observational Routinely Collected Health Data) provides a 21-item checklist to improve transparency and reproducibility of RWE studies [12] - acknowledging that rigor, not design type, determines credibility.

Crucially, evidence pluralism includes *patient and clinician knowledge* as valid forms of evidence. The patient's lived experience - captured through digital diaries, social media, or qualitative interviews - complements quantitative RWD and can reveal outcomes overlooked in traditional metrics (e.g., impact on daily functioning, stigma, or caregiver burden).

Implementing evidence pluralism requires new competencies:

- **Methodological**: Understanding causal inference (e.g., propensity scoring, instrumental variables), data quality assessment, and bias mitigation.
- **Interpretive**: Judging the trustworthiness of RWE sources and the appropriateness of analytical choices.
- **Ethical**: Ensuring patient privacy, data governance, and equitable representation in RWD sources (noting that EHRs and claims data often underrepresent marginalized populations).

Regulators, researchers, and clinicians must move beyond asking "*Is this from an RCT?*" to "*Is this evidence fit-for-purpose, transparently generated, and relevant to my decision?*"

# 1.4. Conclusion

Real-World Evidence is not a replacement for randomized trials but a necessary expansion of the evidence ecosystem. By capturing the messiness, diversity, and dynamism of actual healthcare delivery, RWE answers questions that traditional research cannot. In an era of precision medicine, value-based care, and rapid innovation, integrating RWE into decision-making - guided by rigorous methods, transparent reporting, and a pluralistic view of evidence - is no longer optional. It is foundational to deliver safe, effective, and equitable care for all patients.

## 1.4.1. References

1. U.S. Food and Drug Administration. Framework for FDA's Real-World Evidence Program. Silver Spring, MD: FDA; 2018

2. European Medicines Agency. Guide on real-world evidence provided by EMA: support for regulatory decision-making. Amsterdam: EMA; 152628/2024

3. Ford I, Norrie J. Pragmatic Trials. N Engl J Med. 2016;375(5):454–463.

4. NIH Health Care Systems Research Collaboratory. Pragmatic Clinical Trials Demonstration Projects. Bethesda, MD: National Institutes of Health; 2023.

5. Ball R, Robb M, Anderson SA, Dal Pan G. The FDA's Sentinel Initiative: A comprehensive approach to medical product surveillance. Clin Pharmacol Ther. 2016;99(3):265-8.

6. Berger ML, Sox H, Willke RJ, Brixner DL, Eichler HG, Goettsch W, et al. Good practices for real-world data studies of treatment and/or comparative effectiveness: recommendations from the joint ISPOR-ISPE Special Task Force on real-world evidence in health care decision making. Value Health. 2017 Sep;20(8):1003-8

7. Fleurence RL, Ramsey SD, et al. Assessing Real-World Data From Electronic Health Records for Health Technology Assessment: The SUITABILITY Checklist: A Good Practices Report of an ISPOR Task Force. Value Health. 2024 Jun;27(6):673-81.

8. 21st Century Cures Act, Pub. L. No. 114-255, 130 Stat. 1033 (2016).

9. U.S. Food and Drug Administration. FDA approves new use of transplant drug based on real-world evidence [Internet]. Silver Spring (MD): FDA; 2021 Jul 16

10. National Institute for Health and Care Excellence (NICE). NICE real-world evidence framework [Internet]. London: NICE; 2022 Jun 23 [cited 2026 Jan 5]. Available from: https://www.nice.org.uk/corporate/ecd9/resources/nice-realworld-evidence-framework-pdf-1124017502405.

11. La Caze A. Evidence-Based Medicine Must Be... J Med Philos. 2009;34(5):509–527. doi:10.1093/jmp/jhp034

12. Benchimol EI, Smeeth L, Guttmann A, Harron K, Moher D, Petersen I, et al. The REporting of studies Conducted using Observational Routinely-collected health Data (RECORD) statement. PLoS Med. 2015 Oct 6;12(10):e1001885.

# Chapter 2. What Is Real-World Data?

Real-World Data (RWD) form the bedrock of Real-World Evidence (RWE). Without high-quality, fit-for-purpose RWD, even the most sophisticated analytical methods cannot yield trustworthy insights. Yet "real-world data" is not a monolithic category. It encompasses a diverse *ecosystem of data sources* - ranging from decades-old administrative claims to cutting-edge wearable sensors - each with distinct strengths, limitations, and governance considerations. Understanding this landscape is essential for anyone designing, evaluating, or using RWE.

## 2.1. Definitions and Scope: Primary vs. Secondary RWD

The FDA and EMA define real-world data (RWD) as:

"*data relating to patient health status and/or the delivery of health care routinely collected from a variety of sources*" [1, 2].

Even though EMA provides some examples, the definition deliberately avoids prescribing specific data types, recognizing that RWD evolve with technology and healthcare systems.

However, a useful conceptual distinction exists between primary and secondary RWD:

- **Primary RWD** are collected prospectively with a specific research or regulatory question in mind, though still within routine care settings. Examples include data gathered in observational studies (case report forms), pragmatic clinical trials, de novo patient registries or surveys.
- **Secondary RWD** are collected for purposes which are not related to the research question in mind (e.g., billing, clinical care, public health reporting) and later repurposed for research. Most EHR and claims data fall into this category.

With these definitions, a patient registry is primary data for the research purpose it is established for (*de-novo* registry), and secondary data for all other research which may be conducted based on the already collected data (*secondary use* registry).

This distinction matters because **data provenance** - the origin, context, and intended use of data - directly affects data quality, completeness, and suitability for analysis. Secondary data may lack structured fields for key variables (e.g., disease severity) of the research question, contain coding errors, or omit critical clinical details. Primary RWD, while more curated, may introduce selection bias if enrollment is non-representative, or suffer from recall bias. It also matters with regards to regulations related to patient privacy. For example, in a jurisdiction the collection of primary data would need patient consent whereas the use of secondary data would not under certain conditions.

Critically, neither type is inherently superior. The key criterion is **fitness for purpose**, a principle emphasized by FDA, EMA and ISPE/ISPOR [3-5]. A secondary claims database may be perfectly adequate for assessing hospitalization rates, while a primary registry with validated endpoints may be needed to evaluate nuanced clinical outcomes like functional status or treatment adherence.

# 2.2. Core Sources of Real-World Data

The landscape of RWD can be broadly categorized into traditional clinical systems, administrative databases, and emerging digital health technologies. While traditional sources like Electronic Health Records (EHRs) and Claims databases provide the backbone for most regulatory submissions, the rise of registries and wearable sensors has introduced new dimensions of granularity and continuous monitoring.

Table 2.1 provides a high-level comparison of these core and emerging sources. A detailed analysis of the strengths, limitations, and technical standards for each source follows in the subsequent sections.

## 2.2.1. The "Secondary-First" Strategy

Within the pragmatic constraints of real-world evidence research, a "Secondary-First" approach is often the most rational starting point for an RWE study. This principle dictates that researchers should prioritize the use of existing data sources - such as administrative claims or electronic health records - as long as they satisfy the established fitness-for-purpose criteria. The primary drivers for this strategy are the significantly lower costs and accelerated timelines associated with secondary data, which is already collected and "ready" for curation. If the initial feasibility assessment reveals that secondary data can adequately answer the research question with sufficient reliability and relevance, the substantial burden of primary collection can be avoided.

However, this is not a compromise on quality, but a tiered evaluation. If the existing data is found to be insufficient - perhaps lacking a specific clinical biomarker, a critical patient-reported outcome, or sufficient longitudinality - the strategy must shift. In such cases, the researcher should consider a hybrid approach, augmenting the secondary "backbone" with targeted primary data collection. If the gaps remain too wide to bridge through augmentation, the strategy then mandates a move to primary data collection or a prospective registry upfront. By following this hierarchy, the researcher ensures that the study design remains as efficient as possible, and avoids operational waste, without ever sacrificing the scientific integrity required for regulatory or clinical acceptance.

**Table 2.1 Core sources of real-world data**

| Source | Primary Use | Variables | Strengths | Limitations |
|---|---|---|---|---|
| **Primary Data** | Targeted observational research (Prospective). | Bespoke endpoints, specific biomarkers, lifestyle factors. | High internal validity; investigator control over protocols. | Costly; slower execution; smaller, potentially biased sample |
| **EHRs** | Point-of-care delivery; clinical documentation. | Lab results, vitals, imaging, physician notes, genomics. | High temporal resolution; "unstructured" clinical nuances. | Missingness; fragmented care across vendors. |
| **Claims / Billing** | Insurance, billing & administrative tracking. | ICD/CPT codes, drug costs, hospitalizations, ER visits. | Massive scale; longitudinal history (often 10+ years). | Lacks clinical severity, lab results; reflects billing incentives |
| **Registry** | Specialized disease or product monitoring. | Standardized outcomes, device performance, PROs. | High-quality, curated data; validated for specific research goals. | Selection bias (e.g., academic sites only); high maintenance cost. |
| **Digital / Wearables** | Continuous health & behavior monitoring. | Heart rate, sleep, glucose, gait, real-time activity. | Continuous, objective data captured in natural environment. | Lack of clinical validation; data silos; privacy/ethical concerns. |
| **Surveys / PROs** | Capturing the "Patient Voice" and QoL | Symptoms, functional status, treatment burden. | Direct insight into lived experience without clinician filter. | Recall bias; low adherence rates; "digital divide" |

### 2.2.2. Primary (Prospective) Data

Primary data collection involves gathering information directly for a specific research purpose through observational studies, such as prospective cohorts or non-interventional studies, but it also includes surveys. Unlike secondary RWD, the investigator controls the data collection environment.

- **Strengths:**
    - High internal validity: Data is collected using standardized protocols tailored to the research question.
    - Completeness: Minimizes "missingness" for critical variables (e.g., specific biomarkers or lifestyle factors).
    - Customization: Allows for the inclusion of specific validated PROs or digital endpoints.
- **Limitations:**
    - Cost and time: significantly more expensive and slower than analyzing existing databases.
    - Smaller scale: Usually limited to hundreds or thousands of patients rather than millions.
    - Bias: Patients who agree to participate may differ from the general "real-world" population, and the information submitted could be also subjective (e.g. on drug utilization or adherence).
- **Ideal Use Case:**
    - Validating a new digital biomarker, studying a rare disease where no registry exists, or fulfilling post-marketing safety requirements (PASS) where specific clinical nuances are required.

### 2.2.1. Electronic Health Records (EHRs)

EHRs are digital versions of patients' medical charts, used by clinicians at the point of care. They contain rich clinical information:

diagnoses, medications, lab results, vital signs, imaging reports, clinical notes (often unstructured), and sometimes genomic data.

**Strengths**

- High clinical granularity and temporal resolution
- Capture longitudinal patient journeys across care settings
- Include both structured (e.g., lab values) and unstructured (e.g., physician notes) data
- Great for understanding epidemiology of disease and patient characteristics

**Limitations**

- Data quality varies by institution, specialty, and EHR vendor
- Inconsistent coding (e.g., ICD-10 vs. SNOMED CT) and documentation practices
- Missing data, often not at random, due to patient's clinical conditions (e.g. if overweight then BMI more likely to be recorded), transfers or fragmented care
- Limited capture of health behaviors or social determinants

EHRs are increasingly standardized through initiatives like Fast Healthcare Interoperability Resources (FHIR), an HL7 standard enabling modular data exchange [6]. The OHDSI community has developed the OMOP Common Data Model (CDM), which transforms heterogeneous EHR data into a standardized analytics-ready format used in multinational studies [7].

## 2.2.2. Administrative, Claims and Billing Data

Claims data are generated when healthcare providers submit bills to insurers (public or private). In the U.S., common sources include Medicare (Parts A, B, D), Medicaid, and commercial insurers (e.g., Optum, IBM MarketScan). Internationally, national health systems (e.g., UK's CPRD, Sweden's National Registers, France's Assurance Maladie) provide similar data.

Claims contain coded information on:

- Diagnoses
- Procedures
- Prescribed medications
- Healthcare utilization (hospitalizations, ER visits, outpatient visits)
- Costs and payments

**Strengths**

- Massive scale (millions of patients)
- Longitudinal coverage (often 10+ years)
- Representative of insured populations
- Excellent for tracking utilization, costs, and treatment patterns

**Limitations**

- No clinical details (e.g., lab values, disease severity)
- Coding may reflect incentives rather than clinical reality
- Lack data on over-the-counter drugs, lifestyle, or social determinants
- Cannot capture outcomes not linked to healthcare encounters (e.g., death outside of hospital)

Despite limitations, claims data are widely used in regulatory submissions, comparative effectiveness research, and safety surveillance (e.g., FDA's Sentinel Initiative).

### 2.2.3. Registries

Registries are organized systems that collect uniform data on specified populations, often focused on a disease (e.g., cancer, rheumatoid arthritis), a medical product (e.g., implantable devices), or a procedure (e.g., joint replacement). If a registry is established for the specific research question in mind, it is primary data. If an existing registry is used to answer a new research question it is secondary data.

Registries can be:

- **Disease-based**: e.g., SEER (Surveillance, Epidemiology, and End Results) for cancer or ICGG (International Collaborative Guacher Group registry)
- **Product-based**: e.g., FDA's National Breast Implant Registry or Bupropion Pregnancy Registry in Europe
- **Clinical quality registries**: e.g., American College of Cardiology's PINNACLE

**Strengths:**

- Standardized data collection protocols
- High data quality and validation
- Often include PROs and long-term outcomes
- Designed for specific research or safety questions

**Limitations:**

- May suffer from selection bias (e.g., only academic centers participate)
- Resource-intensive to maintain
- Limited generalizability if enrollment criteria are narrow

The AHRQ recommends clear governance, defined endpoints, data quality and transparency in methodology to maximize utility and improve patient outcomes [8].

## 2.3. Emerging Digital Data Sources: Wearables, Apps, and Sensors

The digital health revolution has expanded RWD beyond traditional healthcare systems. **Wearables** (e.g., *Fitbit*, *Apple Watch*, *Oura ring*), **mobile health apps**, and **biosensors** now generate continuous, objective physiological and behavioral data.

Common data types include:

- Physical activity (steps, active minutes)
- Heart rate and rhythm (including ECG via smartwatches)
- Sleep patterns
- Glucose levels (continuous glucose monitors)
- Respiratory rate and oxygen saturation

**Strengths**

- Real-time, high-frequency measurements
- Capture data in natural environments (not just clinics)
- Enable remote monitoring and early intervention
- Empower patients through data access

**Limitations:**

- Validation: Many consumer devices lack clinical validation; accuracy varies by metric and population
- Representativeness: Users tend to be younger, healthier, and higher-income - introducing selection bias
- Data silos: Proprietary formats and lack of interoperability hinder integration with EHRs

- Privacy and ethics: Continuous monitoring raises concerns about data ownership, consent, and algorithmic bias

Regulatory bodies are adapting. The FDA's Digital Health Center of Excellence provides guidance on software as a medical device (SaMD) and validation of digital endpoints [9].

## 2.4. Patient-Reported Outcomes (PROs) and Patient-Generated Health Data (PGHD)

**Patient-Reported Outcomes (PROs)** are direct reports from patients about their health status, symptoms, function, or quality of life - without interpretation by clinicians [10]. PROs differ from clinician-reported or performance-based outcomes.

**Patient-Generated Health Data (PGHD)** is a broader term encompassing any health-related data created, recorded, or gathered by patients (or caregivers) outside clinical settings. This includes PROs, but also data from apps, journals, home devices, and social media.

Why PROs and PGHD matter:

- Capture the patient's lived experience - often missed in clinical notes
- Inform shared decision-making and person-centered care
- Serve as endpoints in regulatory trials (e.g., FDA's PRO Guidance [10])
- Reveal treatment burden, symptom fluctuations, and unmet needs

Common PRO instruments include:

- *EQ-5D*: A standardized, generic instrument developed by the EuroQol Group to measure health-related quality of life across five dimensions - mobility, self-care, usual activities, pain/discomfort, and anxiety/depression -

with both a descriptive system and a visual analog scale (EQ VAS).

- *PROMIS (Patient-Reported Outcomes Measurement Information System)*: A National Institutes of Health (NIH)-funded suite of computer-adaptive, validated questionnaires that assess physical, mental, and social health domains (e.g., fatigue, pain interference, physical function) using item response theory to minimize respondent burden while maximizing precision.
- Disease-specific tools: Instruments tailored to capture symptoms, function, or quality of life impacts unique to a particular condition. For example, the *Health Assessment Questionnaire (HAQ)* is widely used in rheumatoid arthritis to evaluate a patient's ability to perform daily tasks across eight categories, such as dressing, walking, and hygiene.

These instruments vary in scope - from broad (EQ-5D) to highly contextual (HAQ) - and are selected based on the research question, population, and regulatory or clinical context.

Challenges include:

- Recall bias and subjective interpretation
- Low adherence to repeated surveys
- Lack of standardization across studies
- Digital divide: older or socioeconomically disadvantaged patients may be underrepresented

Best practices from the ISPOR PRO Good Practices Task Force emphasize selecting validated instruments, using electronic PROs (ePROs) to improve compliance, and integrating PROs into routine care workflows [11].

## 2.5. Data Linkage: Connecting the Dots

No single RWD source captures the full spectrum of a patient's health journey. Data linkage - the process of connecting records from different sources that refer to the same individual - enables more comprehensive, powerful analyses.

Common linkage scenarios:

- **EHR + claims:** combine clinical detail with long-term utilization and outpatient drug use
- Registry + EHR: validate registry data with real-time clinical information
- Wearable data + EHR: correlate physiological trends with clinical events

**Linkage methods:**

- *Deterministic*: exact match on identifiers (e.g., name, DOB, SSN). High precision but fails with typos or missing fields.
- *Probabilistic*: statistical matching based on multiple fields (e.g., name, ZIP, sex). More flexible but may introduce false matches.
- *Privacy-preserving (tokenization):* use encrypted tokens or trusted third parties to avoid sharing personally identifiable information (PII).

Key considerations while linking data include:

- **Privacy and ethics**: Linkage often requires explicit patient consent or Institutional Review Board (IRB) waivers. GDPR (EU) and HIPAA (US) impose strict rules on re-identification risk [12].
- **Data quality**: Errors in identifiers lead to mislinkage, biasing results.

- **Governance**: Clear data use agreements and stewardship frameworks are essential.

Successful examples include:

- *UK's Secure Anonymized Information Linkage (SAIL) Databank*, linking primary care, hospital, and mortality records in Wales[13]
- *FDA's Sentinel System*, which links claims and EHR data across multiple data partners for safety surveillance [14]

### 2.5.1. Data Integration and Analytics Platforms

The true power of RWD is realized not through isolated sources, but through the strategic convergence of multiple datasets. Through advanced **data integration and linkage layers**, researchers can bridge the "clinical depth" of EHRs with the "longitudinal breadth" of administrative claims at the individual patient level. These linkages - achieved via deterministic methods (using unique identifiers like Social Security or National ID numbers) or probabilistic methods (using statistical matching of age, sex, and zip codes) - create a holistic view of the patient journey. Once harmonized into a common structure, the integrated data is fed into sophisticated analytics platforms. These platforms utilize a spectrum of methodologies - ranging from traditional biostatistics to machine learning and AI - to transform raw data into insights that address a variety of critical regulatory, market access strategies, healthcare and commercial questions. Figure 2.1 shows a flow diagram of such integration.

## 2.6. Conclusion

Real-World Data are as diverse as the healthcare systems and technologies that generate them. From the structured codes of insurance claims to the continuous streams of wearable sensors, each source offers unique windows into patient health - alongside distinct limitations. The art and science of RWE lie not in seeking a "perfect" data source, but in strategically selecting, combining, and validating RWD to address specific questions with rigor and transparency. As digital health accelerates and regulatory acceptance grows, the RWD landscape will continue to evolve. Researchers and decision-makers must stay grounded in core principles: fitness for purpose, data quality assessment, ethical stewardship, and methodological transparency.

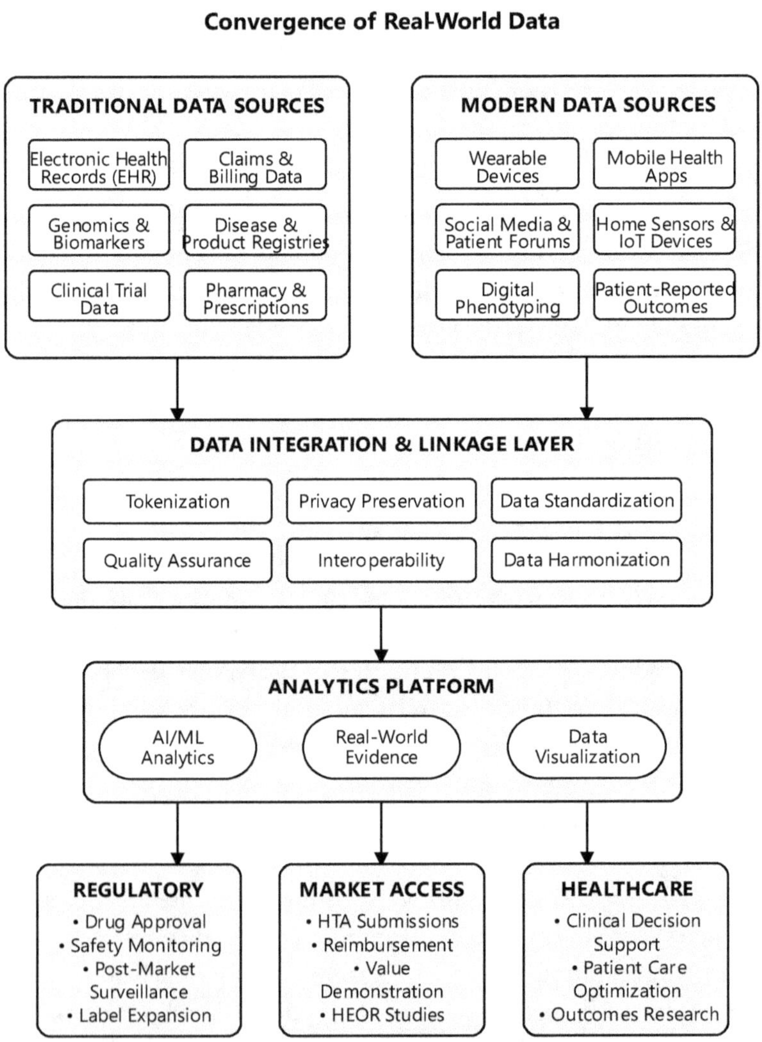


**Figure 2.1 Data Integration and Analytics Platform**

## References

1. U.S. Food and Drug Administration. Framework for FDA's Real-World Evidence Program. Silver Spring (MD): FDA; 2018 Dec.

2. European Medicines Agency. Guide on real-world evidence provided by EMA: support for regulatory decision-making. Amsterdam: EMA; 2024 Jun 20. Report No.: EMA/152628/2024.

3. U.S. Food and Drug Administration. Considerations for the Use of Real-World Data and Real-World Evidence to Support Regulatory Decision-Making for Drug and Biological Products: Guidance for Industry. Silver Spring (MD): FDA; 2023 Aug.

4. European Medicines Agency. Data quality framework for EU medicines regulation. Amsterdam: EMA; 2023 Oct. Report No.: EMA/815001/2021.

5. Gatto NM, Campbell UB, Rubinstein E, et al. A structured process to identify fit-for-purpose data (SPIFD): a scientific guide for the selection of real-world data to support regulatory-quality real-world evidence. Pharmacoepidemiol Drug Saf. 2021;30(S1):147.

6. Health Level Seven International. HL7 FHIR Release 5. Ann Arbor (MI): HL7; 2023.

7. Observational Health Data Sciences and Informatics (OHDSI). The OMOP Common Data Model. New York: OHDSI; 2023.

8. Gliklich RE, Dreyer NA, Leavy MB, editors. Registries for Evaluating Patient Outcomes: A User's Guide. 4th ed. Rockville (MD): Agency for Healthcare Research and Quality (US); 2020 Sep. Report No.: 20(21)-EHC020.

9. U.S. Food and Drug Administration. Digital Health Center of Excellence. Silver Spring (MD): FDA; 2024.

10. U.S. Food and Drug Administration. Guidance for Industry. Patient-reported outcome measures: use in medical product development to support labeling claims. Silver Spring (MD): FDA; 2009.

11. Rothman ML, Belger M, Gater A, et al. Recommendations on patient-reported outcome measure development and selection: a report of

the ISPOR PRO Good Practices Task Force. Value Health. 2022 Jan;25(1):1-15.

12. European Union. Regulation (EU) 2016/679 of the European Parliament and of the Council of 27 April 2016 on the protection of natural persons with regard to the processing of personal data and on the free movement of such data, and repealing Directive 95/46/EC (General Data Protection Regulation). Off J Eur Union. 2016 May 4 [cited 2026 Jan 5];L119:1-88.

13. SAIL Databank. Secure Anonymised Information Linkage (SAIL) Databank. Swansea (UK): Swansea University; c2026.

14. U.S. Food and Drug Administration. Sentinel Initiative. Silver Spring (MD): FDA; 2024.

# Chapter 3. Where RWE Is Used Today

Real-world evidence (RWE) has transitioned from a supportive role to a central engine of evidence generation across healthcare. While randomized controlled trials (RCTs) remain essential for establishing *efficacy* under tightly controlled conditions, RWE - derived from real-world data (RWD) - addresses questions about *effectiveness, safety in diverse populations, value for money,* and *implementation feasibility* in routine care [1]. Increasingly, regulators, clinicians, industry, and payers rely on RWE not as a substitute for RCTs, but as a complementary and often indispensable source of insight.

## 3.1. Pharmaceuticals

Drug development and use have become the most mature domain for RWE, with regulators now routinely accepting real-world data for trial design, external controls, and post-marketing commitments.

### 3.1.1. Expanding the Evidence Continuum

RWE now supports drug development across the entire lifecycle - from early target discovery to post-marketing commitments - and is especially valuable when RCTs are impractical (e.g., in rare diseases or long-term outcomes).

- **Target identification**: Large-scale biobanks linked to electronic health records (EHRs), such as the UK Biobank (500,000 participants), enable researchers to scan thousands of phenotypes for associations with genetic variants [2]. Another example, researchers sequenced biobank participants from five different sources to identify rare "human knockouts" lacking the ANGPTL3 gene. These individuals naturally exhibited lower lipid levels and reduced heart disease risk without adverse effects, validating ANGPTL3 as a safe, effective target for the drug evinacumab [3].

- **Clinical trial design & feasibility**: Before launching a trial, sponsors use RWD to estimate recruitment windows, natural history curves, and background event rates [4,5]. A notable case involved Roche using Flatiron Health's U.S. oncology EHR data to model progression-free survival in metastatic uveal melanoma - a disease so rare that traditional power calculations were highly uncertain - enabling a smaller, faster Phase II trial.

- **External (synthetic) control arms**: In single-arm trials - common for oncology or ultra-rare conditions - RWE can serve as a comparator. The FDA accepted an external control arm constructed from historical EHR and registry data to support the 2020 approval of pembrolizumab for any solid tumour with high microsatellite instability (MSI-H), a tissue-agnostic indication. The control group was carefully matched on histology, line of therapy, and performance status; sensitivity analyses confirmed robustness across multiple data sources [6,7].

- **Post-approval safety monitoring**: Regulators routinely require RWE-based studies following approval. After canagliflozin showed an unexpected signal for lower-limb amputations in the CANVAS RCT, the FDA mandated a large post-marketing study using Medicare claims and commercial databases. This RWE study confirmed the risk and refined it to higher-risk subgroups (e.g., patients with prior amputation or peripheral artery disease), enabling targeted safety communications [8].
- **Utilization research**: RWE provides essential insights into clinical practice, enabling researchers to evaluate patient adherence, long-term persistence, and the real-world impact of risk minimization effectiveness. A classical example is the series of studies conducted to evaluate risk minimization measures related to pregnancy prevention program of valproate, sponsored by a consortium [9-11].

## 3.1.2. Regulatory Harmonization and Transparency

Global regulators now articulate clear expectations for RWE submissions:

- The U.S. FDA's 2023 guidance on RWE for regulatory decision making demands rigorous demonstration of data fitness for use, comparability between RWD and trial populations, and transparent reporting of all analytical decisions - including how missing data and treatment switching were handled [12].
- The European Medicines Agency (EMA) coordinates RWE generation across the EU via DARWIN EU, a distributed research network designed to produce timely, protocol-driven evidence for regulatory questions (e.g., COVID-19 vaccine safety in pregnancy) [13].
- Methodologically, the RWE Transparency Checklist [14] and ISPOR-ISPE Good Practices Report on reproducibility and validity [15] provide field-wide benchmarks for study quality

- particularly around transparency, quality control, outcome validation, and reproducibility.

When proposing an RWE study to regulators, it is recommended to pre-specify the analysis plan in a public protocol (e.g., on ClinicalTrials.gov, or HMA-EMA Catalogue) and commit to publishing both positive and null findings.

## 3.2. Medical Devices

### 3.2.1. A Natural Fit for Real-World Data

Unlike pharmaceuticals, most medical devices evolve quickly, are used heterogeneously, and depend on operator skill - all factors that limit the generalizability of RCTs. RWE, especially from registries and linked claims, often provides more relevant and timely evidence.

- **Pre-market evidence for moderate-risk devices**: Many Class II devices in the U.S. (e.g., orthopaedic implants, certain IVDs) are cleared via the 510(k) pathway providing *substantial equivalence* to a predicate device. FDA encourages using RWD instead of bench testing or clinical trials for these cases and has provided a list of 90 examples in a report [16]. For instance, a novel knee prosthesis was cleared based on 3-year survivorship data from the American Joint Replacement Registry (AJRR), showing non-inferior revision rates to predicate devices in over 15,000 matched patients.
- **Post-market surveillance under EU MDR**: The EU Medical Device Regulation now mandates systematic use of RWE for post-market clinical follow-up (PMCF) [17]. A striking example came from the Netherlands, where the Dutch Arthroplasty Register (LROI) detected a two-fold increase in revision surgeries for a specific dual-mobility hip cup - prompting rapid manufacturer recall and a field safety notice, all within 18 months of market entry [18].
- **Humanitarian and pediatric devices**: For devices targeting small populations - such as the HeartWare HVAD pediatric

ventricular assist device - RWE from compassionate-use programs and international registries (e.g., INTERMACS) formed the bulk of the evidence for FDA humanitarian device exemption (HDE) approval, since RCTs were deemed unethical or infeasible due to very small sample size [19].

### 3.2.2. Methodological Rigor

Key standards now guide device RWE:

- ISO/TR 20916:2019 sets expectations for clinical performance studies of IVDs using RWD, emphasizing analytical validity and traceability of samples [20].
- The FDA's 2022 guidance stresses the need to verify that device identifiers (UDIs) are accurately recorded and linkable to clinical outcomes in claims or EHRs - a non-trivial challenge in fragmented U.S. systems [21].
- The IDEAL-R framework extends the surgical innovation pathway to explicitly incorporate registry-based evidence at each stage (*Idea → Development → Exploration → Assessment → Long-term study*), with iterative learning built in [22].

As an example, the HeartMate 3 LVAD received expanded FDA approval for destination therapy based partly on 2-year RWE from INTERMACS, which showed lower rates of pump thrombosis and disabling stroke compared to earlier-generation devices - even among high-risk patients excluded from the pivotal MOMENTUM 3 RCT [23].

## 3.3. Health Technology Assessment (HTA)

### 3.3.1. Demonstrating Value in the Real World

While regulators focus on safety and efficacy, payers and HTA bodies focus on *value* - specifically, whether a new intervention justifies its cost relative to current standards of care. RWE is now essential for bridging the "evidence gap" between idealized trial results and actual clinical practice.

- **Refining Economic Models:** Payers use RWD to replace hypothetical assumptions in cost-effectiveness models. For instance, instead of using trial-based adherence rates, RWD from pharmacy claims can provide realistic "persistence" data, which often significantly alters the predicted Budget Impact Analysis (BIA) [24].
- **Conditional Reimbursement & Managed Entry:** In many European markets, HTA bodies grant "conditional" coverage for promising but high-cost therapies (like CAR-T cell therapies). This is often contingent on the manufacturer collecting long-term RWE via registries to confirm that the "pivotal" outcomes observed in small trials translate to sustained survival in the broader population [25].
- **Indication Expansion and Pricing:** RWE has been used to support the value proposition for expanding existing drugs into new populations. A landmark case involved the use of RWE to secure reimbursement for palbociclib in male breast cancer, a population too small for traditional Phase III trials, by leveraging clinical outcomes from multiple EHR-based cohorts [26].
- **Performance-Based Risk-Sharing Agreements (PBRSAs):** Innovative contracts are increasingly tied to real-world outcomes. For example, a payer may agree to reimburse a high-cost heart failure medication only if RWE confirms a reduction in the rate of hospitalizations within the first six months of treatment, as tracked through integrated claims data [27]

### 3.3.2. Evolution of Payer Frameworks

National and regional bodies are formalizing how they weigh RWE:

- **NICE (UK):** The National Institute for Health and Care Excellence recently published its *Real-World Evidence Framework*, which outlines how RWE should be used to inform high-quality HTA, emphasizing the need for transparency in data provenance and "fit-for-purpose" data quality [28].

- **G-BA/IQWiG (Germany):** Recent legislation (GSAV) allows the G-BA to mandate RWE collection for orphan drugs at the point of market entry to reduce uncertainty regarding long-term benefit [29].
- **CADTH (Canada):** The Canadian Agency for Drugs and Technologies in Health is increasingly utilizing RWE to monitor the "real-world" performance of oncology drugs, potentially leading to price renegotiations, for example if real-world survival falls below trial-based estimates [30].

# 3.4. Public Health

## 3.4.1. Agility, Equity, and Accountability

Public health operates in fast-moving, population-scale contexts where waiting for RCTs is often impossible. RWE provides actionable intelligence for surveillance, outbreak response, and equity-focused policy.

- **Early outbreak detection**: For example, during the 2022 monkeypox outbreak, the CDC's *National Syndromic Surveillance Program (NSSP)* - which aggregates chief complaints from >7,000 U.S. emergency departments - detected a spike in "rash" and "lesion" visits in major cities days before the first lab-confirmed case, enabling earlier public alerts and resource mobilization [31].
- **Vaccine safety and effectiveness**: When concerns emerged about myocarditis after mRNA COVID-19 vaccination in adolescents, the Vaccine Safety Datalink (VSD) - a collaboration of 9 integrated healthcare systems - rapidly conducted a self-controlled case-series analysis. It confirmed a small but significantly increased risk after dose 2 in males aged 12–17 (14 excess cases per million doses), supporting targeted risk–benefit communication [32].
- **Health equity monitoring**: Analyses of the CMS Chronic Conditions Data Warehouse revealed that Black patients with heart failure with reduced ejection fraction (HFrEF) were

40% less likely than White patients to receive guideline-recommended SGLT2 inhibitors - even after adjusting for insurance, comorbidity, and provider type. This RWE finding spurred CMS and professional societies to launch equity-focused quality improvement collaboratives [22].

- **Policy evaluation**: A difference-in-differences study using state-level death certificate and prescription data found that states expanding Medicaid under the Affordable Care Act saw a 6% greater reduction in opioid overdose deaths over 5 years compared to non-expansion states - providing strong support for Medicaid's role in addiction treatment access [23].

### 3.4.2. Infrastructure and Ethics

Sustainable public health RWE requires investment in **FAIR-compliant data systems** (*Findable, Accessible, Interoperable, Reusable*) and robust governance [33]. Examples include Wales' *SAIL Databank*, which securely links primary care, hospital, and mortality records using privacy-preserving anonymization; and *Singapore's National Electronic Health Record (NEHR)*, which includes opt-out consent and tiered researcher access [34-5]. The WHO's 2023 *Handbook on Real-World Evidence for Public Health* offers a globally adaptable framework, especially for low-resource settings where paper-based systems still dominate [36].

It is to be noted that ecological analyses (e.g., regional vaccination rates vs. case rates) are prone to *ecological fallacy*. Whenever possible, individual-level data and multivariable adjustment should be used, with reporting aligned to the *RECORD statement* [37].

## 3.5. Health Tech and AI

### 3.5.1. Powering the Digital Revolution - Responsibly

Digital health tools and AI algorithms are increasingly deployed in clinical workflows - but their promise hinges on rigorous, real-world validation. RWE is indispensable for training, testing, and monitoring these technologies.

- **Bias detection and mitigation**: An algorithm developed by Optum to predict patient healthcare needs was found - using RWE from multiple U.S. health systems - to systematically underestimate risk for Black patients because it used "past healthcare costs" as a proxy for "health needs". Since Black patients historically had lower access to care (and thus lower costs), the model misclassified many as low-risk. Re-training with direct clinical markers (e.g., HbA1c, creatinine) corrected this bias, illustrating how RWE can uncover and fix real-world inequities [38].
- **Continuous learning systems**: Epic uses its massive RWD repository (over 300 million patients) to train "Transformer" models (like GPT, but for medical events) that learn across hundreds of health systems to predict patient outcomes more accurately than static models - which are based on published research and clinical trials [39].
- **Reimbursement and coverage decisions**: Pear Therapeutics' reSET, a prescription digital therapeutic for substance use disorder, was the first FDA-authorized app. To secure Medicare coverage, the company conducted a post-market RWE study showing that patients using reSET alongside standard care had significantly higher abstinence rates (40% vs. 18%) and lower inpatient admissions over 12 weeks - demonstrating both clinical utility and cost savings [40].

## 3.5.2. Evolving Regulatory Landscapes

Regulators are adapting to the dynamic nature of AI:

- The FDA's **Predetermined Change Control Plan (PCCP)** pathway (2023) allows AI developers to prospectively describe how and when their algorithm will be updated based on RWE triggers - avoiding the need for new 510(k) submissions for minor improvements [41].
- The **EU AI Act (2024)** classifies AI systems intended for medical diagnosis or treatment as "high-risk", requiring

ongoing post-market monitoring using RWD, annual transparency reports, and human oversight [42].

- **Reporting standards** like *SPIRIT-AI* (for trial protocols) and *CONSORT-AI* (for results) now require authors to detail data provenance, preprocessing steps, and performance across subgroups (e.g., by age, sex, race) to ensure reproducibility and fairness [43,44].

These advances come with emerging challenges: "Data drift" - e.g., changes in EHR documentation patterns during the pandemic - can silently degrade AI performance. Leading institutions now deploy *shadow mode* (running AI alongside clinicians without acting on outputs) and *drift detection dashboards* to catch degradation early [45].

# 3.6. Hospital Decision-Making

## 3.6.1. From Dashboards to Learning Systems

Hospitals increasingly use RWE not just for reporting, but for **actionable** decision support - spanning clinical care, operations, procurement, and strategy.

- **Clinical pathway refinement**: At Kaiser Permanente, analysts used EHR-derived RWE to show that delays >3 hours in administering antibiotics after sepsis recognition were associated with a 33% increase in in-hospital mortality. This evidence directly informed a system-wide "*Sepsis 3-Hour Bundle*" initiative, which reduced median time-to-antibiotics from 142 to 58 minutes and saved an estimated 120 lives per year [46].

- **Formulary decisions**: This EHR-based study analyzed nearly 200,000 patients to identify real-world GLP-1 discontinuation. It found that 12-month discontinuation was significantly higher in patients with obesity alone (43%) compared to those with type 2 diabetes (31%), highlighting a critical gap between clinical trial adherence and real-world persistence. [47].

- **Risk stratification for care management**: The widely used **LACE index** (*Length of stay, Acuity of admission, Comorbidities, Emergency department visits*) was derived from a primary cohort and validated using administrative data from >1 million Canadian hospital discharges. Hospitals using LACE-guided discharge planning (e.g., assigning high-risk patients to transitional care nurses) have reported 18–22% reductions in 30-day readmissions [48].
- **Value-based contracting**: Under CMS Bundled Payments for Care Improvement (BPCI), a Midwestern health system used RWE to negotiate risk-adjusted pricing with an orthopaedic implant manufacturer. By demonstrating that their surgeons achieved significantly lower revision rates and shorter lengths of stay with a specific knee system called Attune, they secured a 12% cost reduction - shared as savings with the payer [49].

## 3.6.2. Building Data Maturity

RWE impact scales with an organization's data maturity. According to *AHRQ* , maturity is measured by how an organization moves from using data for *simple reporting* (Level 1) to using data for *robust process improvement* (Level 5), where real-time RWE is used to prevent harm before it happens [50].

Open-source platforms like OHDSI's *OMOP Common Data Model* allow hospitals to standardize data structure and run reproducible RWE studies (e.g., cohort diagnostics, propensity score matching) using shared analytics tools like ATLAS [51].

Table 3.1 outlines the progressive stages of data maturity within healthcare facilities, illustrating how advancing from siloed systems to integrated, interoperable environments enables increasingly sophisticated real-world evidence applications and predictive analytics [52].

**Table 3.1 Data maturity in healthcare facilities**

| Stage | Data Capability | Example RWE Use |
|---|---|---|
| **1. Siloed** | Separate EHR, lab, billing systems | Monthly report: "Total hip replacements this quarter" |
| **2. Integrated** | Internal data linked (e.g., EHR + pharmacy) | Comparative analysis: "Clopidogrel vs. ticagrelor: bleeding events in ACS" |
| **3. Interoperable** | External linkage (e.g., state cancer registry, socioeconomic data) | Predictive model: "30-day readmission risk, incorporating housing instability" |
| **4. Learning Health System** | Embedded analytics, feedback to care teams | Real-time CDS alert: "High sepsis risk - consider lactate + blood cultures" |

## 3.7. Conclusion

RWE is no longer ancillary - it is embedded in the fabric of modern healthcare decision-making. From accelerating drug approvals to detecting device failures, from tracking pandemics to auditing algorithmic fairness, RWE provides the contextual richness that controlled trials cannot. Yet its power is matched by responsibility: poor-quality data, unmeasured confounding, and insufficient transparency can mislead as easily as inform.

The path forward lies in three commitments:

1. **Methodological rigor** - grounded in guidelines like RECORD, STROBE, and the RWE Transparency Checklist
2. **Regulatory collaborations** - as seen in FDA's RWE Framework and EMA's DARWIN EU
3. **Ethical stewardship** - ensuring equity, patient privacy, and public trust.

As data ecosystems converge (EHRs, wearables, genomics, social determinants) and analytical methods advance (e.g., causal machine learning), the potential of RWE will only grow. The challenge - and opportunity - for the next decade is to harness this potential wisely.

## References

1. Sherman RE, Anderson SA, Dal Pan GJ, Gray GW, Gross T, Hunter NL, et al. Real-world evidence - what is it and what can it tell us? N Engl J Med. 2016 Dec 8;375(23):2293-7.

2. Bycroft C, Freeman C, Petkova D, Band G, Elliott LT, Sharp K, et al. The UK Biobank resource with deep phenotyping and genomic data. Nature. 2018 Oct;562(7726):203-9.

3. Dewey FE, Gusarova V, Dunbar RL, O'Dushlaine C, Schurmann C, Gottesman O, et al. Genetic and pharmacologic inactivation of ANGPTL3. N Engl J Med. 2017 Jul 20;377(3):211-21.

4. Evans SR, Paraoan D, Perlmutter J, Raman SR, Sheehan JJ, Hallinan ZP. Real-world data for planning eligibility criteria and enhancing recruitment: recommendations from the Clinical Trials Transformation Initiative. Ther Innov Regul Sci. 2021;55(3):498-507.

5. Dagenais S, Russo L, Madsen A, Webster J, Becnel L. Use of Real-World Evidence to Drive Drug Development Strategy and Inform Clinical Trial Design. Clin Pharmacol Ther. 2022 Jan;111(1):77-89.

6. Marabelle A, Le DT, et al. Efficacy of pembrolizumab in patients with MSI-H/dMMR cancers: Final analysis of the KEYNOTE-164 and KEYNOTE-158 studies. J Clin Oncol. 2020;38(15_suppl):3513.

7. Schmid P, Doi T, et al. Pembrolizumab for MSI-H/dMMR cancers: RWE supporting tissue-agnostic approval. Ann Oncol. 2020;31(1):146–156.

8. Yuan Z, DeFalco FJ, Ryan PB, Stang PE, Berlin JA, Desai M, et al. Risk of lower extremity amputations in people with type 2 diabetes mellitus treated with sodium-glucose co-transporter-2 inhibitors in the USA: A retrospective cohort study. Diabetes Obes Metab. 2018 Mar;20(3):582-589.

9. Toussi M, Bardoulat I, Tcherny-Lessenot S, de Voogd HJ, Dimos V, Kaplan S. Effectiveness of risk minimisation measures for valproate: A cross-sectional survey among physicians in Europe. Pharmacoepidemiol Drug Saf. 2021 Mar;30(3):283-291. doi: 10.1002/pds.5119.

10. Ehlken B, Nishikawa C, Kaplan S, Dresco I, Granados D, Toussi M. Effectiveness of risk minimization measures for valproate: a drug utilization study based on implementation of a risk minimization programme in Europe, analysis of data from the UK. Curr Med Res Opin. 2022 Mar;38(3):461-468.

11. Colas S, Nishikawa T, Kaplan S, Toussi M, et al. Effectiveness of the Additional Risk Minimisation Measures for Valproate Among Healthcare Professionals and Patients: A Cross-Sectional Survey in Six European Countries. Pharmacoepidemiol Drug Saf. 2024. doi: 10.1002/pds.70046.

12. U.S. Food and Drug Administration. Considerations for the use of real-world data and real-world evidence to support regulatory decision-making for drug and biological products: guidance for industry. Silver Spring (MD): FDA; 2023 Aug.

13. Arlett P, Kjaer J, Broich K, et al. Real-world evidence in EU medicines regulation: enabling use and establishing value. Clin Pharmacol Ther. 2022;111(1):21-23.

14. Wang SV, Pinheiro S, Hua W, Arlett P, Uyama Y, Berlin JA, et al. Reporting to improve reproducibility and facilitate validity assessment for healthcare database studies V1.0. Value Health. 2017 Sep;20(8):1009-22.

15. Wang SV, Pinheiro S, Hua W, Arlett P, Uyama Y, Berlin JA, et al. Reporting to improve reproducibility and facilitate validity assessment for healthcare database studies V1.0. Value Health. 2017 Sep;20(8):1009-22.

16. Food and Drug Administration. Examples of Real-World Evidence (RWE) used in medical device regulatory decisions. Silver Spring (MD): FDA; 2021.

17. European Parliament, Council of the European Union. Regulation (EU) 2017/745 of the European Parliament and of the Council of 5 April 2017 on medical devices, amending Directive 2001/83/EC, Regulation (EC) No 178/2002 and Regulation (EC) No 1223/2009 and repealing Council Directives 90/385/EEC and 93/42/EEC. OJ L 117, 5.5.2017, p. 1–175.

18. van Steenbergen LN, van der Linde D, Walstock S, Swierstra BA. Early failure of a dual-mobility hip cup detected by national registry. Acta Orthop. 2015;86(5):530–535.

19. Kirklin JK, Naftel DC, Pagani FD, Kormos RL, Stevenson LW, Blume ED, et al. Seventh INTERMACS annual report: 15,000 patients and counting. J Heart Lung Transplant. 2015;34(12):1495–1504

20. International Organization for Standardization. ISO/TR 20916:2019: In vitro diagnostic medical devices - Clinical performance studies using real-world data. Geneva: ISO; 2019..

21. U.S. Food and Drug Administration. Use of Real-World Evidence to Support Regulatory Decision-Making for Medical Devices. Guidance. 2022.

22. Sedrakyan A, von Elm E, et al. IDEAL-R: A Framework for Real-World Evaluation of Surgical Innovation. Ann Surg. 2020;272(3):410–416.

23. Mehra MR, Goldstein DJ, Cleveland JC, Connors JM, Joseph S, Salerno CT, et al. Two-year outcomes with the HeartMate 3 left ventricular assist device: real-world evidence from the INTERMACS registry. Circulation. 2022;145(10):732–43.

24. Garrison LP Jr, Neumann PJ, Erickson P, Marshall D, Mullins CD, Pashos CL, et al. Using real-world data for coverage and cost-effectiveness decisions: the ISPOR Real-World Data Task Force report. Value Health. 2007;10(5):326-335.

25. Jørgensen J, Hanna E, Kefalas P. Outcomes-based reimbursement for gene therapies in practice: the experience of recently launched CAR-T cell therapies in major European countries. J Mark Access Health Policy. 2020;8(1):1715536.

26. Wedam S, Fashoyin-Aje L, Bloomquist E, et al. FDA Approval Summary: Palbociclib for Male Patients with Metastatic Breast Cancer. Clin Cancer Res. 2020;26(6):1208-1212.

27. Neumann PJ, Chambers JD, Simon CJ, Meckley LM. Risk-sharing arrangements that link payment for drugs to health outcomes are

proving hard to implement. Health Aff (Millwood). 2011;30(12):2329-2337.

28. National Institute for Health and Care Excellence (NICE). Real-world evidence framework. London: NICE; 2022.

29. Institute for Quality and Efficiency in Health Care (IQWiG). Routine practice data for the benefit assessment of drugs: Rapid report A19-43. Cologne: IQWiG; 2020 Jan 10. Report No.: A19-43.

30. Bubela T, McCabe C, Archibald P, Huys I, Faulkner S, Johnston JK, et al. Keeping pace with innovation: Real-world evidence in Canada's health system. Health Policy. 2021;125(10):1324-1331.

31. Centers for Disease Control and Prevention (CDC). National Syndromic Surveillance Program (NSSP) in Action: Monkeypox 2022. MMWR Morb Mortal Wkly Rep. 2022 Aug 12;71(32):1027-1031.

32. Klein NP, Lewis N, Goddard K, et al. Surveillance for Adverse Events After COVID-19 mRNA Vaccination. JAMA. 2021;326(14):1390–1399.

33. Wilkinson MD, Dumontier M, Aalbersberg IJ, Appleton G, Axton M, Baak A, et al. The FAIR Guiding Principles for scientific data management and stewardship. Sci Data. 2016;3:160018.

34. Jones KH, Jones AR, et al. SAIL Databank: A trusted research environment for population data science. Int J Popul Data Sci. 2022;7(2):1–10.

35. Ministry of Health (Singapore). National Electronic Health Record (NEHR) [Internet]. Singapore: MOH; 2024 [cited 2026 Jan 6]. Available from: https://www.moh.gov.sg/e-services/national-electronic-health-record-(nehr

36. World Health Organization. Handbook on real-world evidence for public health: a guide for using real-world data to support public health decision-making. Geneva: World Health Organization; 2023.

37. Benchimol EI, Langan SM, Guttmann A, Azoulay L, Fieldes ME, Jones IT, et al. The REporting of studies Conducted using

Observational Routinely-collected health Data (RECORD) statement. PLoS Med. 2015;12(10):e1001885

38. Obermeyer Z, Powers B, Vogeli C, Mullainathan S. Dissecting racial bias in an algorithm used to manage the health of populations. Science. 2019 Oct 25;366(6464):447-53.

39. Epic Research. Generative medical event models improve with scale: introducing the Cosmos Medical Event Transformer (CoMET). arXiv. 2025.

40. Campbell ANC, Nunes EV, et al. Real-world outcomes of reSET, a prescription digital therapeutic for substance use. J Med Internet Res. 2020;22(10):e21897.

41. U.S. Food and Drug Administration. Predetermined Change Control Plans for AI/ML-Based SaMD. Draft Guidance. 2023.

42. European Parliament, Council of the European Union. Regulation (EU) 2024/1689 of the European Parliament and of the Council of 13 June 2024 laying down harmonised rules on artificial intelligence (Artificial Intelligence Act). OJ L, 2024/1689, 12.7.2024.

43. Liu X, Rivera SC, Moher D, Calvert MJ, Denniston AK; SPIRIT-AI and CONSORT-AI Working Group. Reporting guidelines for clinical trial reports for interventions involving artificial intelligence: the CONSORT-AI extension. BMJ. 2020 Sep 9;370:m3164.

44. Rivera SC, Liu X, Chan AW, Denniston AK, Calvert MJ; SPIRIT-AI and CONSORT-AI Working Group. Guidelines for clinical trial protocols for interventions involving artificial intelligence: the SPIRIT-AI extension. Nat Med. 2023 Jan;29(1):44-53.

45. Wiens J, Saria S, Sendak M, Ghassemi M, Liu VX, Doshi-Velez F, et al. Do no harm: a roadmap for responsible machine learning for health care. Nat Med. 2019 Oct;25(10):1337-40.

46. Liu VX, Fielding-Singh V, Greene JD, Baker JM, Iwashyna TJ, Bhattacharya J, et al. The timing of early antibiotics and hospital mortality in sepsis. Am J Respir Crit Care Med. 2017 Oct 1;196(7):856-63.

47. Do D, Lee T, Peasah SK, Good CB, Inneh A, Patel U. GLP-1 receptor agonist discontinuation among patients with obesity and/or type 2 diabetes. JAMA Netw Open. 2024 May 1;7(5):e2413172.

48. van Walraven C, Dhalla IA, Bell C, Etchells E, Stiell IG, Zarnke K, et al. Derivation and validation of an index to predict early death or unplanned readmission after discharge from hospital to the community. CMAJ. 2010 Apr 6;182(6):551-7.

49. Fisher DA, Parkin D. Advancing patient outcomes and economic value in total knee arthroplasty: the evidence of the ATTUNE Knee System. Raynham (MA): DePuy Synthes; 2019. [White Paper].

50. Hatef E, Scholle SH, Buckley B, Weiner JP, Austin JM. Development of an evidence- and consensus-based Digital Healthcare Equity Framework. JAMIA Open. 2024 Dec;7(4):ooae136.

51. Hripcsak G, Duke JD, et al. Observational Health Data Sciences and Informatics (OHDSI): Opportunities for observational researchers. Stud Health Technol Inform. 2015;216:574–578.

# Chapter 4. The RWE Ecosystem

Real-world evidence (RWE) does not emerge in isolation. It is the product of a dynamic, interdependent **ecosystem** - a network of stakeholders, data sources, technologies, and regulatory - ethical frameworks that collectively enable, validate, and apply evidence derived from real-world data (RWD). Understanding this ecosystem is essential for anyone involved in RWE generation: whether designing a study, interpreting results, or deciding on reimbursement or regulatory action. Unlike the controlled environment of randomized clinical trials (RCTs), RWE draws from messy, heterogeneous, and often fragmented reality - making coordination among ecosystem participants not just helpful but *necessary*.

This chapter maps the RWE ecosystem in four parts: (1) key stakeholders and their roles and incentives; (2) data providers and the evolution of data sources; (3) technology enablers and analytical infrastructure; and (4) the ethical and legal scaffolding that underpins trustworthy RWE. Throughout, we draw on the latest regulatory guidance (FDA, EMA, PMDA, WHO), recent landmark initiatives, and concrete examples to illustrate how the pieces fit together - and where tensions remain.

# 4.1. Stakeholders: Purpose, Perspectives, and Tensions

The RWE ecosystem is driven by stakeholders with distinct mandates, evidence needs, and risk tolerances. Their evolving acceptance of RWE signals both progress and persistent challenges.

## 4.1.1. Regulators

Regulators have moved from cautious exploration to active integration of RWE - especially where RCTs are impractical, unethical, or insufficient to capture long-term or rare outcomes. **U.S. Food and Drug Administration (FDA)**: The *21st Century Cures Act* (2016) catalyzed FDA's RWE Program, culminating in the 2018 *Framework for RWE* [1] and the 2021 *RWE Guidance for Drug Developers* [2]. The landmark 2020 approval of pembrolizumab for tumor-agnostic use in MSI-H/dMMR cancers was partially supported by RWE from Flatiron Health's oncology EHR database - one of the first cases where RWE substituted for a confirmatory RCT [3]. In 2023, FDA issued draft guidance on *Using RWE to Support Label Expansions for Approved Drugs*, reaffirming its commitment to RWE in post-marketing settings [4].

- **European Medicines Agency (EMA)**: EMA's approach is more consensus-driven. The *Big Data Steering Group* (2016–2021) laid groundwork, followed by the 2022 *Reflection Paper on RWE for Regulatory Decision-Making* [5], which distinguishes between *confirmatory* (e.g., label extensions) and *exploratory* uses. Notably, the 2022 conditional approval of vutrisiran (for hereditary transthyretin amyloidosis) relied partly on external control arms derived from natural history registries - a precedent for ultra-rare diseases [6].
- **Japan's PMDA & WHO**: Japan's *Sakigake* designation and the *Next Generation Health Database Japan* initiative foster RWE use in aging populations [7].
- **WHO**, The World Health Organization's recent HTA frameworks emphasize pragmatic evidence collection in resource-limited settings, specifically advocating for mobile Health

(*mHealth*) data to evaluate treatment adherence and outcomes where traditional electronic records are unavailable - e.g., using SMS messages in Kenya to assess antiretroviral treatment adherence [8].

Interestingly, regulators are not monolithic. Within agencies, divisions (e.g., oncology vs. rare disease) have divergent comfort levels with RWE - often dictated by disease urgency, data maturity, and precedent. A "*regulatory sandbox*" mindset is increasingly adopted: *iterative dialogue*, *pilot submissions* (e.g., FDA's RWE Pilot Program), and *co-development of protocols*. Table 4.1 provides a few examples of such regulatory sandbox programs.

**Table 4.1 Examples of regulatory sandbox**

| Sandbox Name | Entity | Focus Area |
|---|---|---|
| **AI Airlock** | MHRA (UK) | Testing AI as a Medical Device (AIaMD) in real NHS settings before full market authorization. |
| **AI Regulatory Sandbox** | EU AI Act | A mandatory requirement for EU member states to allow high-risk AI testing under supervision. |
| **CNIL Sandbox** | CNIL (France) | Focuses on data protection (GDPR) for digital health innovators using complex patient datasets. |
| **Telemedicine Sandbox** | MOH (Singapore) | Tested mobile medicine and remote monitoring before the formal licensing laws were even written. |

## 4.1.2. Payers & HTA Bodies

Payers prioritize **value** - comparative effectiveness, cost-effectiveness, and budget impact in routine care. RWE helps answer: *Does this work here, for our patients, at this price?*

- **NICE (UK)** launched its *RWE Programme* in 2021 and published a *Methods Framework* in 2023, requiring RWE studies to meet standards for transparency, bias adjustment, and generalizability [9]. In its appraisal of **semaglutide for obesity**, NICE explicitly requested

RWE on long-term weight maintenance beyond trial duration - a gap RCTs could not fill.

- **Germany's G-BA** (Gemeinsamer Bundesausschuss) accepts RWE in *early benefit assessments* (NUB procedures), notably for **gene therapies** (e.g., Zolgensma), where 5-year RWE commitments offset uncertainty [11].
- **France's HAS** formalized RWE use in its 2023 *Methodological Guide for HTA*, emphasizing real-world comparative effectiveness and data representativeness [40]. In the 2024 reassessment of **fremanezumab for migraine**, HAS accepted SNDS data (national linked claims and hospital records) to evaluate 12-month treatment persistence and resource use - complementing trial evidence [41].
- **ICER (U.S.)** integrates RWE via its *Open-Source Value Project*, using claims and EHR data to model real-world adherence and discontinuation - critical for chronic therapies like PCSK9 inhibitors.

As compared to regulators, payers typically demand longer follow-up and broader populations. This causes tension in the ecosystem as a drug may be *approved* based on RWE but *not reimbursed* if RWE fails to demonstrate real-world durability or equity.

## 4.1.3. Pharmaceutical & Biotech Industry

Industry is both a generator and consumer of RWE - using it for trial design (e.g., synthetic control arms), post-marketing commitments (PMS), life-cycle management, and market access.

- **Trial optimization**: RWE is often used for the identification of the eligible population for clinical trials, or to help finding eligible patients in the right centers. AstraZeneca used Flatiron EHR data to refine inclusion criteria for the **FLAURA2 trial** in EGFR-mutant NSCLC, reducing recruitment time by 30% [12].

- **Post-authorization (post-marketing) safety studies (PASS/PMS)**: This is one of the areas sponsors use RWE traditionally. The use of secondary data has become the default option, an approach known as "secondary first". Sanofi's RWE study of **dupilumab in atopic dermatitis** (using U.S. claims + EHR) satisfied FDA's post-marketing requirement on herpes zoster risk - completed in 18 months vs. projected 5 years for a prospective cohort [13].

Sponsor-led RWE faces perception biases ("marketing data"). Mitigation strategies include pre-specification (e.g., publishing analysis plans on ClinicalTrials.gov), independent steering committees, and open-data collaborations and consortia (e.g., **OHDSI's AstraZeneca–Janssen–Novartis partnership** on diabetes outcomes).

### 4.1.4. Clinicians & Patients

Frontline providers and patients are increasingly *co-creators* of RWE - not just data sources.

- **Clinicians** use RWE for point-of-care decisions (e.g., **PCORnet's hypertension decision support tool**, trained on 10M+ EHR records). But data fatigue and EHR interoperability gaps remain barriers [14].
- **Patient groups** advocate for RWE that reflects patient-reported outcomes (PROs) and quality of life. The **MyHeart Counts** Apple ResearchKit app - which collected activity and symptom data from >50,000 users - demonstrated feasibility of patient-generated RWE [15].

However, clinicians value context (e.g., social determinants), but most RWD lack granularity on lifestyle, environment, or functional status. Structured PRO integration (e.g., PROMIS in EHRs) is a promising frontier.

**Box 4.1: Stakeholder Alignment Checklist**

Before launching an RWE study, ask:

- *Regulators*: Is the study objective aligned with a defined regulatory decision context?
- *Payers*: Does the comparator reflect standard of care in this jurisdiction?
- *Pharma*: Can fit-for-purpose data be found in an existing data source?
- *Clinicians*: Are endpoints clinically meaningful (not just statistical)?
- *Patients*: Were outcomes co-selected? Is data burden minimized?

# 4.2. Data Providers: Diversity, Quality, and Evolution

RWD is the fuel of the RWE engine. Its sources have exploded in volume and variety - but not uniformly in quality or accessibility.

**Table 4.2: Traditional real-world data sources**

| Source | Strengths | Limitations | Example Use |
|---|---|---|---|
| **Electronic Health Records (EHRs)** | Rich clinical detail, longitudinal, point-of-care capture | Variable coding, missing data, limited social context | FDA's Sentinel Initiative for vaccine safety [16] |
| **Administrative Claims** | Large scale, standardized billing codes, longitudinal coverage | Lack clinical nuance, coding for reimbursement ≠ diagnosis | ICER's cost-effectiveness models for GLP-1 RAs [17] |
| **Registries** | High-quality, standardized phenotyping, often PRO-linked | Selection bias, limited generalizability | EMA's use of the *EUROCAT registry* for congenital anomaly monitoring [18] |

### 4.2.1. Traditional sources

The traditional sources of RWD are summarized in table 5. They include electronic health records (EHRs), administrative and reimbursement records, and registries.

### 4.2.2. Emerging Linked Sources

Other sources of data are emerging thanks to the new data sources and possibility of linking them together as mentioned before. More of these linked data sources will become available thanks to technology and methods improvement.

- **Genomics + EHR Integration**: The **All of Us Research Program** (U.S.) links WGS data with EHRs for >350,000 participants - enabling RWE on pharmacogenomics (e.g., CYP2C19 and clopidogrel response) [19].
- **Wearables & Digital Biomarkers:** Apple Heart Study (419,000 participants) detected atrial fibrillation via irregular pulse notifications - a real-world validation of a digital endpoint [20]. FDA's **Digital Health Center of Excellence** now evaluates such data for regulatory use.
- **Social Determinants of Health (SDOH) Data**: U.S. CMS mandates SDOH screening (Z-codes); integrated with EHRs, they helped quantify how housing instability doubled hospital readmission risk in heart failure patients [21].
- **Patient-Generated Data (PGD)**: Apps like MyTherapy track medication adherence; aggregated (anonymized), they revealed 42% non-adherence to oral anticoagulants - far higher than trial reports [22].

### 4.2.3. Data Quality & Fitness-for-Use

"*Garbage in, gospel out*" remains a risk. The **FAIR principles** (Findable, Accessible, Interoperable, Reusable) are now baseline expectations [23]. More critically, **fitness-for-purpose** must be assessed *per study objective*:

For example, for a rare disease prevalence estimate, claims data may be "fit" despite low sensitivity - because high specificity reduces false positives. But for dose-response analysis, EHR clinical notes (NLP-extracted) may be superior.

### 4.2.4. Global Data Landscapes

- **EU**: The European Health Data Space (EHDS), adopted in 2024, mandates secondary use of EHR data for research, with standardized FHIR APIs and citizen consent portals [24].
- **U.S.**: The 21st Century Cures Act Final Rule (2023) prohibits information blocking - accelerating EHR data liquidity, albeit unevenly.
- **LMICs**: Rwanda's TRACnet (HIV treatment database) and India's National Digital Health Mission (NDHM) show how lightweight, mobile-first systems can generate high-impact RWE where infrastructure is limited [25].

## 4.3. Technology Vendors: Enablers and Innovators

RWE's analytical complexity demands robust infrastructure. The translation of raw RWD into actionable RWE relies on a sophisticated - and rapidly consolidating - technology landscape. Vendors no longer serve separate functions; instead, they occupy interlocking roles across the RWE value chain, from data curation to causal inference.

This ecosystem can be usefully categorized into three functional tiers: **data aggregators**, which standardize and enrich heterogeneous sources; **analytics platforms**, which enforce methodological rigor through common data models and reproducible workflows; and **AI/ML specialists**, which extract novel signals while increasingly embedding causal principles.

Table 4.2 outlines representative players and strategic priorities within each tier.

**Table 4.2 Tiers of technology and data vendors**

| Tier | Role | Key Players | Innovation Focus |
|---|---|---|---|
| **Data Aggregators** | Curate, clean, link RWD | IQVIA, Flatiron, COTA, OM1 | Oncology-specific ontologies; real-world genomics |
| **Analytics Platforms** | Standardize analysis | OHDSI (open-source), DataVant, Komodo | Common data models (OMOP, PCORnet), bias diagnostics |
| **AI/ML Specialists** | Extract signals, predict outcomes | Google Health AI, Tempus, Owkin | Federated learning, NLP for clinical notes, synthetic data |

## 4.3.1. Common Data Models (CDMs): The Interoperability Backbone

The **OMOP CDM** (Observational Medical Outcomes Partnership), stewarded by OHDSI, is now used in >30 countries. Its strength: *same code, same meaning*. A 2023 multi-national study used OMOP to harmonize 12 databases (U.S., UK, France, Japan) to assess SGLT2 inhibitor safety - cutting analysis time from 18 months to 6 weeks [26].

Albeit a large step ahead, CDMs don't solve *semantic heterogeneity*. For example, "hypertension" in one EHR may mean diagnosis code; in another, it's a nurse's note. NLP pipelines (e.g., cTAKES, Amazon Comprehend Medical) bridge this - but require local validation.

## 4.3.2. Federated Analytics: Privacy-Preserving Collaboration

Instead of pooling data, federated systems run code *where data resides*. The **EU's EHDEN project** linked 15+ hospitals without data leaving local servers - used for RWE on antibiotic resistance [27]. Similarly, **Trials.ai** (by Unlearn.AI) creates **digital twins** of control arms using federated learning across pharma partners.

### 4.3.3. AI and Causal Inference

Deep learning excels at pattern recognition (e.g., retinal scans predicting CVD risk [28]), but RWE demands causal answers. Vendors now embed causal frameworks:

- **Target Trial Emulation** [29]: Aetion's platform automates emulation design - including eligibility, treatment initiation, and censoring rules.
- **G-Methods** (e.g., IPTW, G-estimation): OHDSI's *CohortMethod* R package includes built-in diagnostics for positivity and covariate balance.

## 4.4. Ethical and Legal Context: Trust as Infrastructure

RWE's legitimacy rests on ethical and legal compliance - especially as data becomes more granular and predictive.

### 4.4.1. Core Principles

- **Autonomy & Consent**: GDPR (EU) and HIPAA (U.S.) differ fundamentally. GDPR requires *explicit, granular consent* for secondary research (Art. 6, 9) unless covered by public interest (e.g., pandemic response). HIPAA permits use of de-identified data without consent - but de-identification standards (Safe Harbor vs. Expert Determination) are contested [30].
- **Justice & Equity**: RWD often underrepresents minorities, rural populations, and LMICs. The **NIH UNITE Initiative** (2021) mandates equity impact assessments for RWE studies using federal data [31]. For example, a 2023 study found voice-based Parkinson's detection models trained on U.S. data failed in Nigerian cohorts due to accent and co-pathology differences [32].

- **Privacy-Utility Trade-off**: Synthetic data (e.g., **Syntegra, MDClone**) can preserve statistical properties while removing identifiers. FDA's 2024 *Synthetic Data Guidance* accepts it for exploratory analyses - but not confirmatory submissions [33].

### 4.4.2. Landmark Regulations & Frameworks

The legal and ethical governance of RWE is shaped by a patchwork of regional frameworks - each reflecting distinct societal values around privacy, public health, and innovation. While no single global standard exists, key regulations increasingly converge on principles of transparency, purpose limitation, and data subject rights. Critically, newer instruments (e.g., the EU's EHDS, updated U.S. health data rules) go beyond protection to enable responsible data reuse - establishing governance pathways, technical standards, and oversight mechanisms specifically for RWE generation. The table below highlights pivotal regulations and their direct implications for RWE practice.

**Table 4.3. Major regulatory landmarks**

| Region | Regulation | Key RWE Impact |
|---|---|---|
| **EU** | GDPR + EHDS Regulation (2024) | Standardized EU-wide data access committees; "data altruism" opt-in for research [24] |
| **U.S.** | 21st Century Cures Act (2016) + FTC Health Breach Rule (2023 update) | Bans data blocking; extends HIPAA-like rules to health apps [34] |
| **Global** | CIOMS Guidelines (2023 update) | Emphasizes community engagement in LMIC RWE studies [35] |

### 4.4.3. Emerging Challenges

- **Algorithmic Bias**: An RWE study using EHR data to allocate kidney transplants was found to disadvantage Black patients due to legacy eGFR equations - prompting FDA's 2023 review of race-correction in diagnostics [36].

- **Commercialization of Data**: When a pharma company licenses a hospital's EHR data, who benefits? The

*Swedish National Data Service* model - where revenue funds public health research - offers one equitable approach [37].

- **Dynamic Consent**: Platforms like *Consent2Share* let participants adjust permissions over time (e.g., "allow cancer research, not mental health"). Piloted in the UK Biobank + NHS integration [38].

## 4.5. Conclusion

The RWE ecosystem is no longer nascent - it is operational, yet fragile. Its strength lies in collaboration: regulators co-developing protocols with industry; clinicians embedding PROs in workflows; patients shaping research questions; and technologists building open, auditable tools.

Yet fragmentation persists. Data silos remain. Analytical standards are adopted unevenly. And trust - especially among marginalized communities - must be continuously earned, not assumed.

The next frontier is not just *more* RWE, but *better* RWE: prospective, diverse, causally rigorous, and ethically grounded. As one EMA advisor put it: *"RWE isn't the alternative to RCTs - it's the reality check."* [39]

### References

1. U.S. Food and Drug Administration. Framework for FDA's Real-World Evidence Program. Silver Spring, MD: FDA; 2018 Dec.

2. FDA. Real-World Evidence: Assessing Electronic Health Records and Medical Claims Data to Support Regulatory Decision-Making for Drug and Biological Products. Guidance for Industry. 2021.

3. Beaver JA, et al. FDA Approval of Pembrolizumab for MSI-H/dMMR Solid Tumors: Implications for RWE. Clin Cancer Res. 2020;26(19):5075–5079.

4. FDA. Using Real-World Evidence to Support Labeling Changes for Approved Drugs and Biological Products. Draft Guidance. 2023.

5. European Parliament, Council of the European Union. Regulation (EU) 2024/1689 of the European Parliament and of the Council of 13 June 2024 laying down harmonised rules on artificial intelligence (Artificial Intelligence Act). OJ L, 2024/1689, 12.7.2024.

6. European Medicines Agency. Amvuttra: EPAR - Public assessment report. Amsterdam: EMA; 2022 Jul 21. Report No.: EMA/CHMP/689555/2022.

7. Pharmaceuticals and Medical Devices Agency. Basic principles on utilization of registry data for new drug application. Tokyo: PMDA; 2021 Mar 23.

8. World Health Organization. Health technology assessment of medical devices. 2nd ed. Geneva: WHO; 2024.

9. NICE. Real-World Evidence: Methods Framework. 2023.

10. Health Canada. Real-World Evidence for Regulatory Decision-Making. 2021.

11. G-BA. Early Benefit Assessment of Gene Therapies: Methodological Considerations. 2022.

12. AstraZeneca. FLAURA2 Trial Design Optimization Using Real-World Data. Press release. 2021.

13. Sanofi. Post-Marketing RWE Study of Dupilumab Safety. ClinicalTrials.gov NCT04565752. 2022.

14. PCORnet. Hypertension Control Initiative: EHR-Based Decision Support. JAMA Intern Med. 2023;183(4):401–410.

15. Perez MV, et al. Large-Scale Assessment of a Smartwatch to Identify Atrial Fibrillation. N Engl J Med. 2019;381:1909–1917.

16. Platt R, et al. The FDA Sentinel Initiative - An Electronic Public Health Surveillance System. N Engl J Med. 2018;378:1565–1567.

17. ICER. GLP-1 Receptor Agonists for Chronic Weight Management. 2022.

18. EUROCAT. Guide 1.4: Registration and Surveillance of Congenital Anomalies. 2021.

19. All of Us Research Program Investigators. The "All of Us" Research Program. N Engl J Med. 2019;381:668–676.

20. Perez MV, Mahaffey KW, Hedlin H, et al. Large-Scale Assessment of a Smartwatch to Identify Atrial Fibrillation. N Engl J Med. 2019;381(20):1909-1917.

21. CMS. CY 2024 Physician Fee Schedule Final Rule. 2023.

22. Arden M, et al. Real-World Adherence to Oral Anticoagulants: Insights from Digital Tracking. J Med Internet Res. 2022;24(7):e36421.

23. Wilkinson MD, et al. The FAIR Guiding Principles. Sci Data. 2016;3:160018.

24. European Commission. Regulation (EU) 2024/xxx on the European Health Data Space. 2024.

25. Binagwaho A, et al. Strengthening Health Systems with Digital Tools: Rwanda's TRACnet Experience. BMJ Glob Health. 2022;7:e008912.

26. Hripcsak G, et al. Multinational Validation of SGLT2 Inhibitor Safety Using OMOP. Lancet Digit Health. 2023;5(11):e784–e794.

27. EHDEN Consortium. Federated Analysis of Antibiotic Resistance Across Europe. PLoS One. 2023;18(4):e0283421.

28. Poplin R, et al. Prediction of Cardiovascular Risk Factors from Retinal Fundus Photographs. Nat Biomed Eng. 2018;2:158–164.

29. Hernán MA, Robins JM. Using Big Data to Emulate a Target Trial. Am J Epidemiol. 2016;183(8):751–758.

30. Office for Civil Rights (HHS). De-identification of PHI. 2022.

31. NIH. UNITE Initiative: Advancing Equity in Biomedical Research. 2021.

32. Oyewole OO, et al. Cross-Cultural Validation of Voice-Based Parkinson's Detection. NPJ Digit Med. 2023;6:142.

33. FDA. Use of Synthetic Data in Regulatory Submissions. Draft Guidance. 2024.

34. FTC. Health Breach Notification Rule Final Amendment. 2023.

35. CIOMS. International Ethical Guidelines for Health-Related Research. 10th ed. 2023.

36. FDA. Review of Race-Based Clinical Algorithms. Internal Report. 2023.

37. Swedish National Data Service. Data Access and Revenue Model. Annual Report. 2023.

38. Kaye J, et al. Dynamic Consent: A Patient Interface for 21st Century Research. Eur J Hum Genet. 2023;31:476–483.

39. EMA Scientific Advice Working Party. Meeting Minutes, Q3 2024. Personal communication.

40. Haute Autorité de Santé. *Guide méthodologique sur l'usage des données du monde réel dans les évaluations médico-économiques*. 2023.

41. HAS. *Avis de la Commission de la transparence – Fremanezumab (Ajovy)*. 28 mars 2024. Avis N° 2024.0056/AS.

# Part II: Study Designs and Methods

# Chapter 5. The RWE Study Lifecycle

The lifecycle of a real-world evidence (RWE) study - from conception to dissemination - differs meaningfully from that of a randomized controlled trial (RCT), yet it demands equal, if not greater, methodological rigor. Unlike RCTs, where design elements are tightly controlled prospectively, RWE studies are shaped by the constraints and sometimes opportunities inherent in clinical practice, or pre-existing data sources. A disciplined, iterative approach is essential to ensure the validity, transparency, and utility of findings for decision-making by regulators, payers, clinicians, and patients. This chapter outlines the four core stages of the RWE study lifecycle - from research question to protocol, data extraction, analysis, and interpretation - with emphasis on practical implementation, methodological trade-offs, and alignment with current regulatory expectations across major jurisdictions.

# 5.1. Study Conception

## 5.1.1. Formulating the Research Question

Formulating a scientifically sound and decision-relevant research question is the critical first step in any RWE study. In contrast to explanatory RCTs, where the aim is often causal inference under idealized conditions, RWE studies typically address *effectiveness*, *safety in routine care*, *disease epidemiology*, *drug utilization* or *healthcare resource use* - questions that require consideration of heterogeneity in populations, settings, and care pathways. The *PICO* (*Population*, *Intervention*, *Comparator*, *Outcome*) framework remains widely used, but for RWE it is often extended to **PICOT-S** (adding *Time* and *Study design*) [1]. However, a well elaborated research question is not necessarily a good one. The **FINER** (*Feasible*, *Interesting*, *Novel*, *Ethical*, *Relevant*) is suggested for spotting good questions [1-2]. The **SPIDER** (*Sample*, *Phenomenon of Interest*, *Design*, *Evaluation*, *Research type*) criteria is suggested as an alternative to PICOT-S for qualitative and mixed-methods contexts [3].

## 5.1.2. Defining the Estimand

Formulating a precise estimand - the precise treatment effect to be estimated - ensures alignment between the clinical question, study design, and statistical analysis. The ICH E9(R1) estimand framework, originally developed for randomized trials, has been adapted for RWE to address a critical vulnerability: ambiguous handling of intercurrent events (e.g., treatment discontinuation, rescue medication, death) that can distort effect interpretation [4]. An estimand is defined by five attributes that collectively specify what is being estimated. Table 5.1 provides the definitions of these attributes applied to an example related to the study comparing GLP-1 RA versus DPP-4 inhibitors for HbA1c reduction.

The choice of intercurrent event strategy fundamentally shapes the estimand's meaning. In the example above, a treatment policy strategy (including post-discontinuation outcomes) estimates effectiveness under routine care conditions - appropriate for payer decisions.

By contrast, a hypothetical strategy (excluding outcomes after discontinuation) estimates the effect if patients remained adherent - more relevant for understanding drug pharmacology but requiring strong assumptions in RWE where adherence is rarely random.

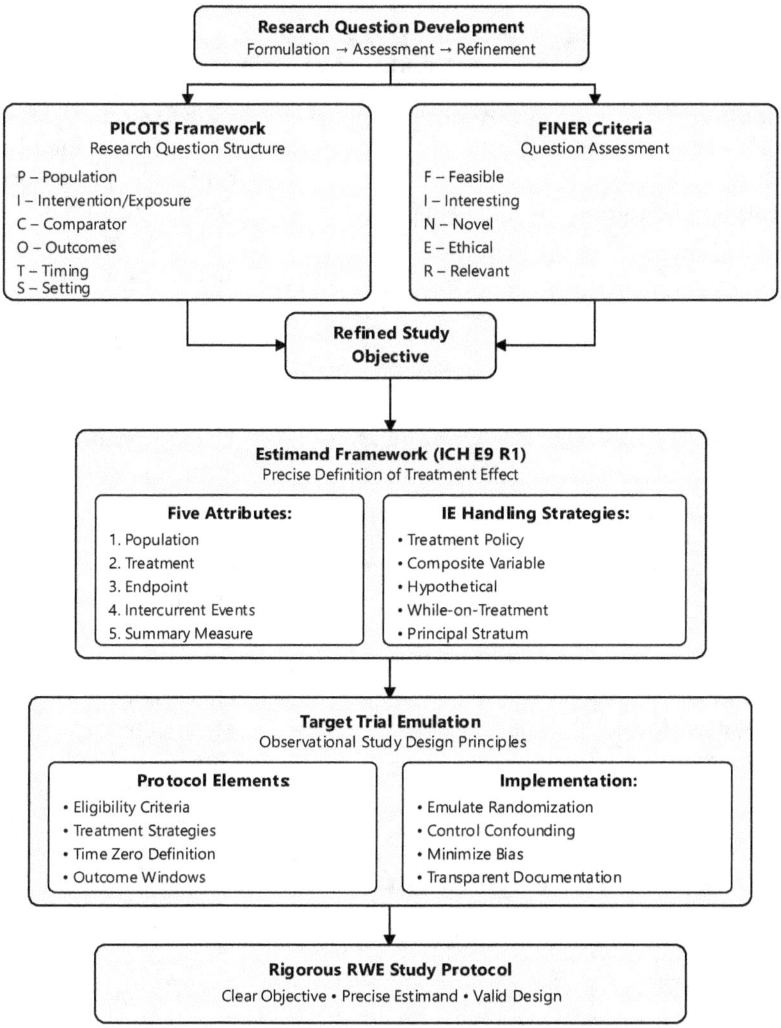


**Figure 5.1. RWE study conception workflow**

Explicitly declaring the estimand a priori prevents post-hoc reinterpretation of results and ensures the analysis plan directly addresses the decision context (e.g., regulatory approval vs. formulary placement). Regulatory agencies now expect estimand specification in RWE protocols supporting label expansions, particularly when intercurrent events are frequent.

**Table 5.1. Attributes of an Estimand**

| Attribute | Description | RWE Example: GLP-1 RA vs. DPP-4 inhibitor for HbA1c reduction |
|---|---|---|
| **Treatment condition** | Intervention and comparator | Semaglutide 1 mg weekly SC vs. sitagliptin 100 mg daily oral |
| **Population** | Target patient group | Adults with T2D, BMI ≥30, HbA1c 7.5–10%, no prior GLP-1/DPP-4 use |
| **Variable** | Outcome measure | Change in HbA1c (%) from baseline to 6 months |
| **Handling of intercurrent events** | Strategy for events affecting interpretation | Treatment policy: Include HbA1c values after discontinuation or rescue therapy to reflect real-world effectiveness |
| **Population-level summary** | Effect metric | Mean difference in HbA1c change (semaglutide minus sitagliptin) |

## 5.1.3. Target trial emulation

A growing number of RWE studies are conducted within *target trial emulation* frameworks - where the protocol is designed to emulate the design elements of a hypothetical pragmatic RCT, including eligibility criteria, treatment strategies, outcome ascertainment windows, and analytic approaches [5]. This paradigm helps align RWE objectives with causal inference principles and improves comparability across studies. A widely cited example is the emulation of the E2100 randomized trial of first-line therapy for HER2-negative metastatic breast cancer, in which real-world data were used to recreate the trial comparing paclitaxel alone with paclitaxel plus bevacizumab; when eligibility criteria, time zero, treatment strategies, and follow-up were aligned with the original protocol, the target trial emulation reproduced a very similar hazard ratio and the same clinical conclusion of only modest overall survival benefit from adding bevacizumab, providing narrower confidence intervals than the RCT, implying more precise estimates [6].

As shown in , target trial emulation (TTE) provides a conceptual scaffold that translates the design logic of a pragmatic randomized trial into an observational analysis plan, thereby strengthening causal inference in RWE. Rather than mimicking an RCT's mechanics, TTE explicitly defines *what* hypothetical trial would answer the research question - and then implements each design element within real-world data constraints. The approach proceeds by mapping five core trial components to observational counterparts:

- **Eligibility criteria**: Define the *target population* using data-derived inclusion/exclusion rules (e.g., "adults with newly diagnosed type 2 diabetes, HbA1c ≥7.5%, no prior insulin") while addressing prevalent-user bias via washout periods or new-user designs
- **Treatment initiation**: Specify a precise *time zero* (e.g., first prescription fill date) and emulate randomization through eligibility assessment at that moment, avoiding immortal time bias
- **Treatment strategy**: Distinguish *initiation* (start of therapy) from *adherence* or *discontinuation*; define grace periods for gaps in exposure and handle treatment switching via *intention-to-treat* or *per-protocol* strategies
- **Outcome ascertainment**: Pre-specify outcome ascertainment windows (e.g., "MACE within 2 years of time zero") with algorithms validated against clinical gold standards
- **Censoring rules**: Define administrative end dates, loss to follow-up criteria, and how competing events (e.g., death from other causes) affect time-at-risk

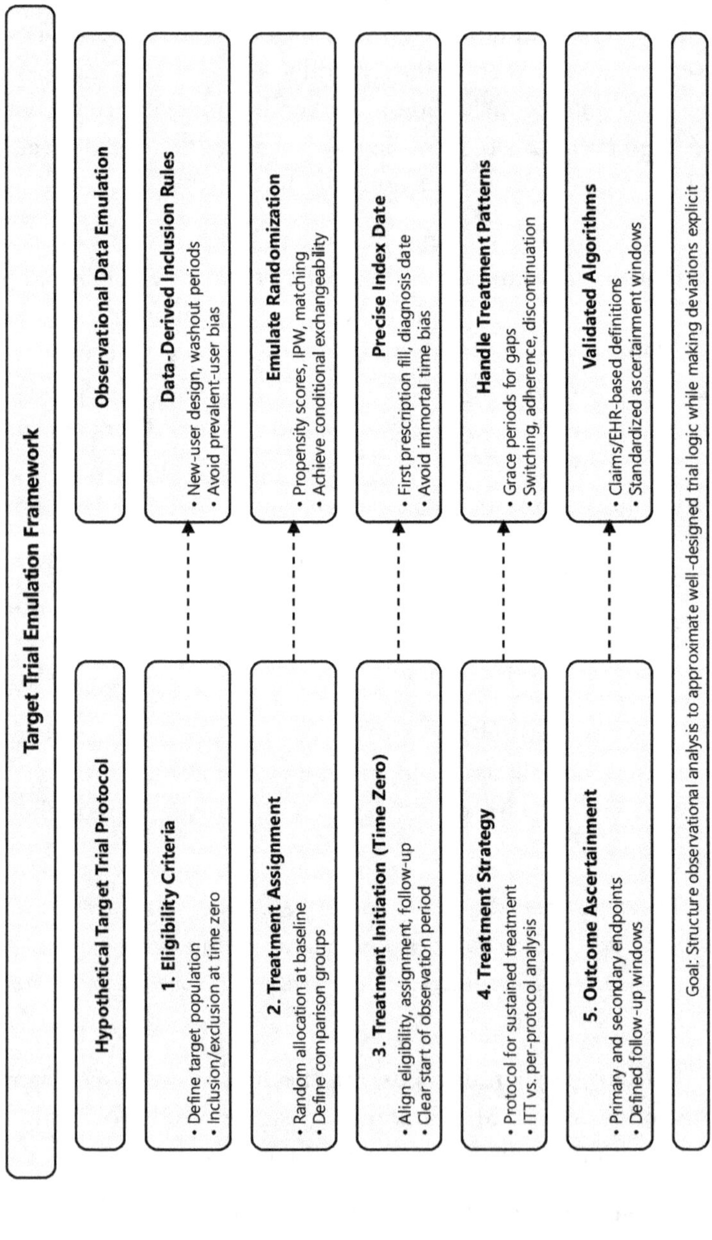


**Figure 5.2. Target Trial Emulation Framework**

By forcing explicit decisions about each design element *before* analysis, TTE minimizes *ad hoc* choices that introduce bias and enhances transparency for regulators evaluating causal claims . Critically, TTE does not guarantee unbiased estimates - it merely structures the analysis to approximate a well-designed trial's logic while making deviations (e.g., unmeasured confounding) explicit and quantifiable through sensitivity analyses.

It is to be noted that estimand and target trial emulation frameworks are not applicable to all RWE studies. They are mostly relevant when the study aims to ascertain the effect of an intervention such as a treatment, an operation, a public health intervention, or a device.

## 5.2. Protocol Development

The research question must be translated into an operational protocol that prespecifies analytic choices while acknowledging the need for exploratory flexibility - particularly where data quality or availability is uncertain.

The key components of an RWE study protocol are presented in Box 5.1. A robust RWE protocol should include:

- A clearly articulated objective and hypothesis (if applicable);

**Box 5.1. Key components of an RWE study protocol**

1. Title and Study ID
2. Version Control and Date
3. Background and Rationale (including policy/clinical decision context)
4. Objectives and Hypotheses
5. Study Design (e.g., cohort, case-control, self-controlled case series)
6. Data Sources (name, version, time coverage, linkage mechanism, validation status)
7. Study Population
    - Inclusion/exclusion criteria
    - Strategies to address immortal time bias, prevalent user bias
8. Exposure, Comparator, and Outcome Definitions
    - Phenotype algorithms (e.g., ICD-10 + ≥2 prescriptions + echocardiography report NLP terms)

- Positive/negative control outcomes for validation

9. Covariates and Confounding Assessment
   - List of measured confounders
   - Plan for unmeasured confounding (e.g., E-value calculation, sensitivity analyses)
10. Statistical Analysis
    - Primary and secondary analyses
    - Model specifications (e.g., Cox with IPTW, marginal structural models)
    - Handling of time-varying exposures and censoring
    - Pre-specified sensitivity and subgroup analyses
11. Ethical and Legal Compliance
12. Timeline, Roles, and Dissemination Plan

- Specification of the target and study populations, including inclusion/exclusion criteria and strategies for handling selection bias (e.g., new-user design, active comparator, prevalent-user washout);
- Definition of exposure, comparator, and outcome variables - including algorithms for phenotyping (e.g., diagnosis codes + medication + lab thresholds for identifying heart failure);
- Description of the data source(s), including provenance, structure, completeness, and validation status; Analytic plan covering covariate selection, confounding control (e.g., propensity score methods, outcome regression, instrumental variables), sensitivity analyses, and handling of missing data;
- Governance and ethical considerations, including data access approvals and patient privacy safeguards compliant with GDPR, HIPAA, or other relevant legislation [7-8].

## 5.2.1. Standardized Protocol Templates for RWE

To operationalize the components of a protocol consistently across studies and jurisdictions, harmonized protocol templates have emerged as essential tools for enhancing reproducibility and regulatory alignment. The HARmonized Protocol Template to Enhance Reproducibility (HARPER), developed through a joint ISPE/ISPOR Task Force consensus process, provides a structured backbone for hypothesis-evaluating RWE studies that use secondary data sources.

HARPER delineates core versus context-specific protocol elements, reducing ambiguity in scientific decisions while accommodating study-specific adaptations for data source characteristics, therapeutic areas, or regulatory contexts [9].

Complementing HARPER, the Structured Template for planning and Reporting on the implementation of Real-World Evidence studies (STaRT-RWE) offers a practical framework focused on implementation fidelity - ensuring that the analytic plan specified *a priori* is executed transparently and that deviations are documented [10].

The study design graphical depiction which is widely known as STaRT-RWE framework diagram (even if this is not exactly its name) offers a useful way to illustrate the design features of an RWE in a readable and precise format.

An example is shown in Figure 5.3.

Both templates explicitly incorporate target trial emulation principles, mandate pre-specification of negative/positive control analyses, and align with FDA and EMA expectations for protocol registration and public availability. Notably, regulatory agencies have begun referencing these templates in guidance documents: the European Network of Centres for Pharmacoepidemiology and Pharmacovigilance (ENCePP) endorses HARPER as a foundation for PASS protocols [11].

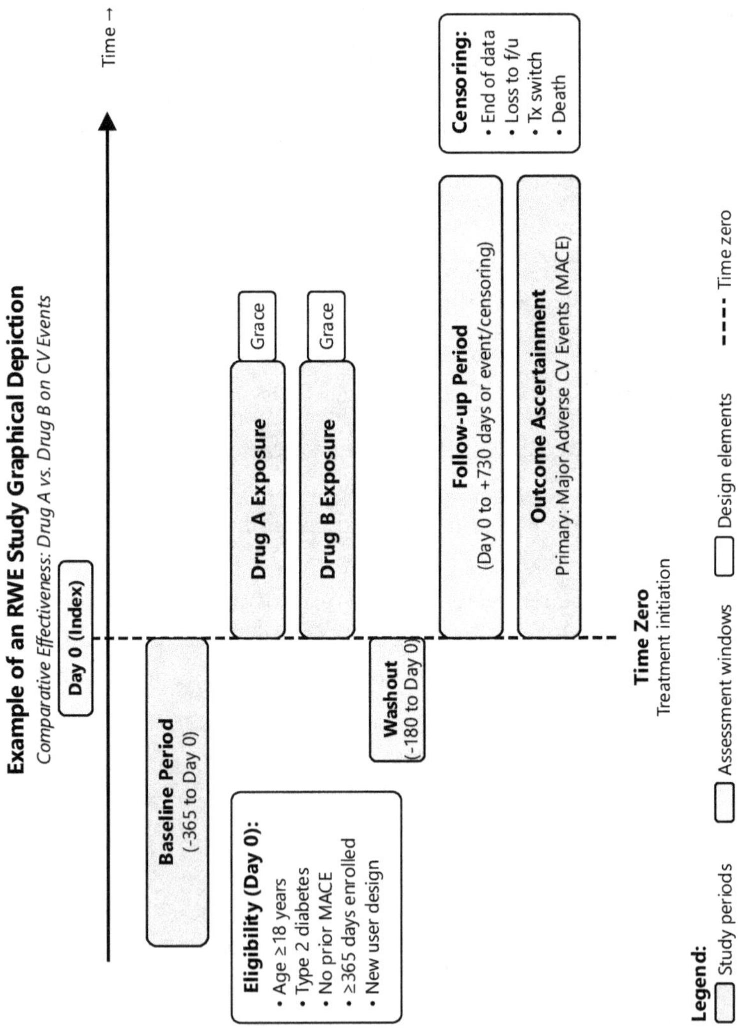


**Figure 5.3 Graphical Depiction of An RWE Study**

Adoption of such standardized templates not only streamlines protocol development but also facilitates cross-study comparability, systematic appraisal by regulators, and independent replication - cornerstones of credible RWE generation.

## 5.2.2. Transparency in protocol development

Regulatory agencies now strongly encourage or require that the study details are defined as *a priori* in a submitted protocol to avoid *a posteriori* modification of study objectives based on the observed results. This is even more important when the study is conducted based on secondary data. FDA emphasizes transparency regarding data collection and analysis in its guidance for the use of RWD and RWE to support regulatory decision-making. It encourages early engagement with FDA using appropriate regulatory pathways, along with the submission of the draft protocol and statistical analysis plan (SAP) [12]. The European Medicines Agency (EMA), requires registration of mandatory post authorization safety study (PASS) protocols and encourages the registration of other protocols to foster transparency [13]. Finally, the International Council on Harmonisation (ICH) encourages researchers to make the study protocol publicly available in appropriate public registers (e.g., ClinicalTrials.gov, the HMA-EMA Catalogue of real-world data studies, or other registers where available) to improve transparency, to support scientific exchange, and to allow the conduct of reproducible research, even where not mandated by regulatory requirements [14].

Rigorous documentation of study protocols is essential for fostering transparency and ensuring the reproducibility of research findings. By explicitly addressing critical methodological components - such as population source eligibility, exposure and outcome algorithms, and confounding assessment strategies - researchers can minimize ambiguity and facilitate external validation. As detailed in Table 5.2, each element of the study design requires specific documentation, ranging from data dictionaries and phenotype definitions to analysis code skeletons and regulatory cross-references. This structured approach not only clarifies decisions regarding design selection and follow-up strategies but also strengthens scientific integrity by allowing peers and regulators to scrutinize the underlying logic and execution of the study. Recent templates such as HARPERR facilitate this documentation.

**Table 5.2. RWE Study Protocol Documentation Checklist**

| Item | Questions to Address | Documentation Requirement |
|---|---|---|
| **Population source** | Which database(s) or registries? What are inclusion/exclusion criteria? | Data dictionary, eligibility algorithm (SQL/OMOP CDM) |
| **Exposure definition** | New-user vs. prevalent? Duration, dose, adherence metric? | Exposure algorithm, validation report (PPV, sensitivity) |
| **Outcome definition** | Incident vs. prevalent? Validation status? | Phenotype definition (e.g., PheKB, OHDSI), adjudication plan |
| **Design selection justification** | Why cohort vs. case–control? Power calculation? | Sample size justification (e.g., *powerSurvEpi* R package) |
| **Control selection (if applicable)** | Matching factors? Sampling strategy (risk-set, density)? | Matching algorithm, balance diagnostics (standardized mean differences) |
| **Follow-up strategy** | Start/stop rules? Handling of loss to follow-up? | Censoring rules, sensitivity analysis plan |
| **Confounding assessment** | Which baseline and time-varying covariates? Planned adjustment method (PS, MSM, g-formula)? | Covariate list, DAG (directed acyclic graph) figure, PS model specification |
| **Statistical analysis plan** | Primary estimator (HR, OR, PR)? Model diagnostics? | Analysis code skeleton, reproducibility statement (e.g., GitHub repo) |
| **Regulatory alignment** | Does the design meet FDA RWE Framework or EMA guidance? | Cross-reference to relevant sections of guidance documents |

## 5.3. Data Extraction

Data extraction in RWE is not a mechanical process but a *knowledge-intensive translation* of clinical and operational reality into analyzable variables. The fidelity of this translation determines the internal validity of the entire study. While RCTs collect data via standardized case report forms, RWE relies on heterogeneous sources -prospectively collected data, electronic health records (EHRs), claims databases, registries, patient-reported outcomes, and increasingly, linked multi-source ecosystems (e.g., EHR + genomics + wearables). Each source introduces distinct challenges related to structure (structured vs. unstructured), coding practices (e.g., ICD-10 vs. SNOMED CT), granularity (visit-level vs. longitudinal), and temporal alignment.

A systematic approach to secondary data extraction and validation comprises three phases [15]:

- **Conceptual mapping / phenotype definition:** Clinical and methodological experts collaboratively define the target constructs (e.g., "incident diabetes") in terms of measurable data elements. Phenotypes (clinical conditions of interest) are defined and used to build "target outcome cohorts".
- **Operationalization:** Those constructs are operationalized into executable algorithms - often involving combinations of diagnosis codes, procedure codes, laboratory values, free-text terms (via natural language processing), and temporal rules (e.g., "first HbA1c ≥6.5% after ≥2 prior normal values").
- **Validation:** the algorithm is validated against a gold standard, typically manual chart review, curated reference sets, or a high-fidelity registry, yielding positive predictive value (PPV), sensitivity, and specificity estimates. Table 5.3 provides an overview of typical validation approach per data source type in the context of their strengths and limitations.

**Table 5.3. Typical validation approach for common data source types**

| Data Source | Strengths | Key Limitations | Typical Validation Approach |
|---|---|---|---|
| **Claims (e.g., Medicare, HIRA)** | Large scale, longitudinal, linked to enrollment/demographics; strong for utilization & cost | No clinical detail (e.g., labs, vitals); coding for billing ≠ clinical reality; lag in submission | PPV via chart review; comparison with registries (e.g., SEER-Medicare linkage) [16] |
| **EHRs (e.g., UK CPRD, US Epic/EPIC-derived CCAE)** | Rich clinical detail; labs, vitals, notes; real-time capture | Fragmented across systems; variable data entry practices; missing structured fields | Feasibility pilot + PPV for key phenotypes; NLP validation against expert annotation |
| **Disease Registries (e.g., SWEDEHEART, NCDR)** | High clinical fidelity; standardized collection; audit trails | Limited generalizability; selection bias; narrow scope | Internal consistency checks; linkage to national death registries for outcome validation [17] |
| **Patient-Generated Data (e.g., Apple Heart Study, MyHeart Counts)** | Captures behavior, symptoms, adherence in naturalistic settings | Self-selection bias; variable device accuracy; high attrition | Calibration against clinic-measured endpoints; sensitivity analysis by engagement level [18] |

Several large-scale initiatives have advanced best practices in this area.

- The U.S.-based **Observational Health Data Sciences and Informatics (OHDSI)** community has standardized the *Common Data Model* (CDM), enabling harmonization of disparate databases (e.g., IBM MarketScan, Optum, CPRD) into a unified schema - OMOP CDM - where exposures, outcomes, and covariates are mapped to standard vocabularies [19].

- In Europe, the **European Health Data & Evidence Network (EHDEN)** has adopted OMOP and built a federated infrastructure allowing distributed analytics without raw data sharing, complying with GDPR's data minimization principle [20].
- Building on this infrastructure, the EMA's **Data Analysis and Real World Interrogation Network (DARWIN EU)** became fully operational in 2024, providing a central platform for rapid, multi-country RWE studies across Europe using a federated network of data partners [21].
- **Japan's Medical Data Vision (MDV)** database similarly uses a standardized structure aligned with claims and receipt data, facilitating national safety studies [22].

Crucially, data extraction must account for temporal dynamics. For time-to-event analyses, misalignment of index dates (e.g., prescription fill vs. dispensation vs. actual ingestion) can introduce bias. Likewise, outcome misclassification is often time-dependent: a stroke coded at initial presentation may later be reclassified as a transient ischemic attack after imaging. Dynamic phenotyping - where algorithm thresholds adapt based on data recency or source reliability - can improve accuracy [23]

Missingness is ubiquitous in RWE data and rarely completely at random. For example, body mass index (BMI) is frequently missing in claims but variably recorded in EHRs; its absence may correlate with patient frailty or primary care engagement. Rather than automatic imputation, researchers should first characterize missingness patterns (e.g., using missingness maps) and assess implications for bias. Sensitivity analyses using multiple imputation, pattern-mixture models, or complete-case restrictions with inverse probability weighting are recommended [24].

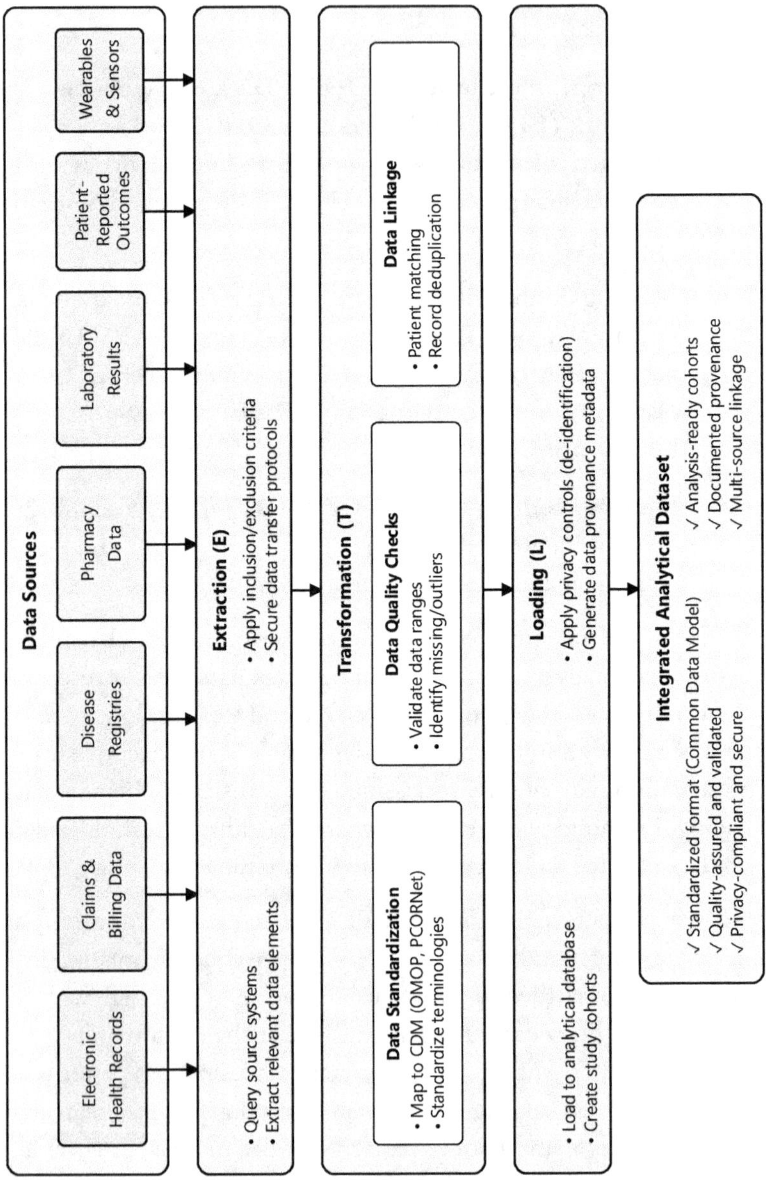


**Figure 5.4. Data extraction pipeline for a multi-source RWE Study**

## 5.4. Analysis

The analytical phase transforms curated data into evidence - but not all statistically significant findings constitute *credible* evidence. RWE analyses must confront three interrelated challenges: *confounding*, *time-related biases*, and *model dependency*. Unlike RCTs, where randomization balances measured and unmeasured confounders (on average), observational analyses rely on measured covariates and structural assumptions to approximate causal effects. Consequently, analytical choices must be justified not only statistically but *epistemologically* - i.e., in terms of the underlying data-generating process.

A tiered analytical strategy is recommended:

1. **Descriptive analyses** to characterize populations, exposure patterns, outcome incidence, and balance of covariates;
2. **Primary causal analysis** using methods aligned with the study design and data structure;
3. **Robustness checks** to assess sensitivity to assumptions and unmeasured confounding.

For hypothesis evaluating studies, common approaches include:

- **Propensity score methods**: Matching, stratification, inverse probability of treatment weighting (IPTW), or covariate adjustment. IPTW is preferred when estimating marginal (population-average) effects, but requires careful trimming and diagnostics (e.g., standardized mean differences <10%, overlap plots) [25].
- **Outcome regression models** (e.g., Cox, logistic) with rich covariate adjustment - increasingly using high-dimensional propensity scores or machine learning-derived confounder summaries [26].
- **Marginal structural models (MSMs)** for time-varying treatments and confounding, using stabilized IPTWs to handle treatment switching or dose escalation [27].

**Box 5.2. Checklist for transparent RWE analysis reporting**

☐ Pre-specified primary and sensitivity analysis models
☐ Full covariate list with coding and handling of missingness
☐ Propensity score diagnostics (balance plots, overlap assessment)
☐ Handling of time-at-risk (e.g., grace periods, exposure lag)
☐ Approach to censoring (e.g., loss to follow-up, administrative end)
☐ Negative/positive control results
☐ E-value or other quantitative bias analysis
☐ Code and data documentation sufficient for independent replication
☐ Compliance with reporting guidelines (e.g., REporting of studies Conducted using Observational Routinely-collected Data [RECORD])

Self-controlled designs (e.g., self-controlled case series [SCCS], case-crossover) offer protection against time-invariant confounding by using each individual as their own control. The SCCS, for instance, compares event rates during risk windows (e.g., 0–42 days post-exposure) to control windows (e.g., >90 days pre- or post-exposure). This method powered the rapid safety signal detection for myocarditis after mRNA COVID-19 vaccines in the UK and US [28-9].

Increasingly, **negative and positive control analyses** are embedded within the primary analysis plan. A negative control is an exposure-outcome pair with no plausible causal link (e.g., statins and wrist fracture); observing an association suggests residual bias. A positive control is a known association (e.g., NSAIDs and GI bleeding); failure to detect it suggests outcome misclassification or insufficient power [30].

Tools like *empirical calibration* (e.g., using the R package *EmpiricalCalibration*) adjust p-values and confidence intervals based on the observed null distribution from negative controls [31].

Finally, *reproducibility* must be engineered into the analysis. Containerization (e.g., Docker), version-controlled code (e.g., GitHub), and executable notebooks (e.g., R Markdown, Jupyter) ensure auditability.

## 5.5. Interpretation

Interpretation is where scientific evidence meets decision-making - and where overconfidence can be most damaging. The goal is not merely to report an effect estimate and p-value, but to contextualize it within the *totality of evidence*, the *study's limitations*, and the *decision environment* in which it will be used.

Three principles guide credible interpretation:

1. **Honesty about uncertainty:** Uncertainty extends beyond confidence intervals. Systematic uncertainty - stemming from unmeasured confounding, outcome misclassification, or selection bias - often dwarfs random sampling error. The E-value provides a quantitative threshold: the minimum strength of association that an unmeasured confounder would need with both exposure and outcome to explain away the observed result [32]. For example, in a study reporting HR (hazard ratio) = 1.8 (95% CI (confidence interval): 1.4–2.3) for a drug and acute kidney injury, the E-value is 2.7 - meaning any unmeasured confounder would need to be associated with both exposure and outcome by a risk ratio of at least 2.7 to nullify the finding. If plausible confounders (e.g., severity of underlying illness) are unlikely to meet that threshold, confidence in causality increases.

2. **Distinction between association and causation:** Language matters. Phrases like "X is associated with Y" are appropriate when causal assumptions are weak; "X may increase the risk of Y" signals tentative causality; "X causes Y" should be reserved for settings where bias is convincingly ruled out (e.g., consistent findings across robust designs, biological plausibility, dose–response).

3. **Transparency about generalizability:** Generalizability - external validity - must be explicitly addressed. An RWE study conducted in a single integrated delivery system (e.g., Kaiser Permanente) may not reflect outcomes in fee-for-service settings or low-resource countries. Analysts should describe the causal contrast (e.g., "effect of initiating Drug A vs. Drug B among commercially insured U.S. adults aged 40–75 with type 2 diabetes and no prior CVD") and avoid overextrapolation. Tools like transportability weighting can

formally adjust estimates to a target population (e.g., national Medicare beneficiaries) when covariate distributions differ [30].

Finally, interpretation should be framed for the intended audience. For regulators, emphasize alignment with the evidentiary standard for the decision (e.g., "substantial evidence" of effectiveness under FDCA §505(b)(2)); for clinicians, highlight absolute risk differences and number needed to treat/harm; for patients, discuss trade-offs in understandable terms (e.g., "For every 100 people treated, 3 fewer will be hospitalized, but 1 may experience side effect Z").

A landmark example is the 2021 FDA approval of **aducanumab** for Alzheimer's disease, supported in part by RWE on real-world diagnostic patterns and treatment pathways. While the pivotal RCTs showed conflicting results, RWE helped characterize the natural history of biomarker-positive early Alzheimer's and the feasibility of implementing amyloid PET/MRI monitoring in routine practice - context essential for benefit–risk assessment, though not for establishing efficacy per se [34]. This illustrates a critical nuance: RWE often strengthens *indirect* evidence (e.g., disease understanding, feasibility) even when direct causal inference remains uncertain.

**Credible interpretation of real-world evidence demands systematic appraisal across multiple dimensions of validity - not merely statistical significance. The C.A.U.T.I.O.N. mnemonic depicted in**

Box 5.3 operationalizes this discipline by requiring explicit assessment of confounding (measured and unmeasured via E-values), algorithm validity (PPV/sensitivity), time-related biases, internal validity checks (negative/positive controls), and alignment of outcomes with clinical decision contexts [33]. Through this multi-faceted scrutiny researchers can honestly contextualize effect estimates within their systematic uncertainties and avoid overconfident causal claims.

**Box 5.3. Framework for Interpreting RWE: The C.A.U.T.I.O.N. Mnemonic**

**C**onfounders assessed? (Measured and unmeasured)
**A**lgorithm validity confirmed? (PPV, sensitivity for key variables)
**U**ncertainty quantified? (CI, E-value, sensitivity analyses)
**T**ime biases addressed? (Immortal time, time-lag, calendar effects)
**I**nternal validity supported? (Negative/positive controls, replication)
**O**utcome relevance established? (Clinically meaningful, decision-aligned)
**N**arrative consistency? (With RCTs, biology, prior RWE)

## 5.6. Reporting

Beyond analytical transparency, the credibility of RWE hinges on comprehensive, standardized reporting that enables critical appraisal and replication. The **STrengthening the Reporting of OBservational studies in Epidemiology (STROBE)** statement established foundational principles for observational research reporting [35], but its generic structure left gaps for RWE-specific challenges such as data provenance, phenotype validation, and handling of time-varying confounding in secondary data.

To address these limitations, the **REporting of studies Conducted using Observational Routinely-collected health Data (RECORD)** extension was developed as a STROBE supplement, adding 13 items specific to routinely collected data - including explicit documentation of data source characteristics (e.g., coding systems, linkage methods), variable derivation algorithms, and missingness patterns [36]. The **RECORD-PE** extension further refines reporting expectations for pharmacoepidemiology studies, by recommending a more granular reporting of the study design, study entry criteria, exposure, fitness for use of the data sources, and confounding control [37]. Adoption of these structured reporting templates not only supports regulatory expectations but also elevates scientific discourse - enabling systematic reviewers to assess risk of bias consistently and allowing clinicians to gauge the applicability of findings to their practice settings. Ultimately, rigorous reporting transforms raw statistical output into interpretable evidence fit for decision-making.

## 5.7. Educational material and applied tools

For readers seeking to apply these methodological principles interactively, the companion **EvidenceMastery™** platform is accessible via the QR code provided at the outset of this volume. Beyond supplementary educational resources, the platform hosts an integrated suite of AI-augmented tools designed to streamline the real-world evidence development lifecycle and improve its education.

- **ConceptAi™ and ProtocolAi™** facilitate the generation of study concept documents and draft protocols through the input of a research question or structured PICOTS parameters.
- **FeasibilityAi™** enables rigorous evaluation of operational feasibility and systematic data landscape characterization.
- **SAPAi™** allows users to automatically derive a comprehensive statistical analysis plan, including table shells specific to the study. The analytical workflow then proceeds to **CodeAi™**, which generates executable statistical programming code customized to the user's preferred language and data model architecture.
- **ReportAi™** and **ManuscriptAi™** transform analytical outputs into structured study reports and subsequently convert finalized reports into publication-ready manuscripts.

Consistent with prevailing regulatory guidance, these AI-augmented tools are designed to operate under a human-in-the-loop principle and should be regarded primarily as educational and performance enhancement resources. Notwithstanding this designation, structured user surveys to date indicate that expert-supervised workflows leveraging these tools consistently yield outputs of scientific quality that are equivalent to, and in several methodological domains, superior to, those produced through conventional expert-driven processes. Collectively, these tools were developed by the author to operationalize the frameworks detailed in this volume and its subsequent publications, systematically integrating established regulatory and methodological guidelines with advanced artificial intelligence capabilities.

## 5.8. Conclusion

The RWE study lifecycle is not linear but cyclical: interpretation often reveals gaps that prompt new questions, refined phenotypes, or enriched data collection - feeding the next iteration. As data ecosystems grow richer and analytical methods more sophisticated, the imperative remains unchanged: **rigor, transparency, and humility**. The most impactful RWE studies are those that acknowledge their limitations while contributing a well-defined piece to the evolving mosaic of evidence - guiding decisions that improve real-world health outcomes.

### References

1. Hulley SB, Cummings SR, Browner WS, Grady DG, Newman TB. Designing Clinical Research. 4th ed. Lippincott Williams & Wilkins; 2013.

2. Fandino W. Formulating a good research question: Pearls and pitfalls. Indian J Anaesth. 2019;63(8):611-616.

3. Cooke A, Smith D, Booth A. Beyond PICO: the SPIDER tool for qualitative evidence synthesis. Qual Health Res. 2012;22(10):1435–1443.

4. International Council for Harmonisation of Technical Requirements for Pharmaceuticals for Human Use (ICH). E9(R1) training material: estimands and sensitivity analysis in clinical trials. Geneva (CH): ICH; 2022.

5. Hernán MA, Robins JM. Causal Inference: What If. Boca Raton: Chapman & Hall/CRC; 2020.

6. Dickerman BA, García-Albéniz X, Logan RW, et al. Emulating a randomized trial of first-line therapies for metastatic breast cancer using real-world data. J Natl Cancer Inst. 2023;115(8):1020-1030.

7. European Union. Regulation (EU) 2016/679 of the European Parliament and of the Council of 27 April 2016 on the protection of

natural persons with regard to the processing of personal data and on the free movement of such data (General Data Protection Regulation). Official Journal of the European Union. 2016;L119:1-88.

8. U.S. Department of Health and Human Services. Guidance on HIPAA Privacy Rule and Sharing of PHI for Research. 2022.

9. Wang SV, Pottegård A, Crown WH, et al. HARmonized Protocol Template to Enhance Reproducibility of hypothesis-evaluating real-world evidence studies on treatment effects: a good practices report of a joint ISPE/ISPOR task force. Value Health. 2022;25(10):1663-1672.

10. Wang SV, Schneeweiss S, Berger ML, et al. Reporting to improve reproducibility and facilitate validity assessment for healthcare database studies: Structured Template for Planning and Reporting on the Implementation of Real-World Evidence Studies (STaRT-RWE). Pharmacoepidemiol Drug Saf. 2021;30(9):1117-1131.

11. ENCePP. Guide on Methodological Standards in Pharmacoepidemiology. Rev 4. EMA/384741/2022.

12. U.S. Food and Drug Administration. Considerations for the use of real-world data and real-world evidence to support regulatory decision-making for drug and biological products: guidance for industry. Silver Spring (MD): FDA; 2023 Aug.

13. European Medicines Agency (EMA). Guideline on good pharmacovigilance practices (GVP): Module VIII - Post-authorisation safety studies (Rev 3). Amsterdam (NL): EMA; 2017.

14. International Council for Harmonisation; European Medicines Agency, Committee for Medicinal Products for Human Use (CHMP). ICH M14 guideline on general principles on planning, designing, analysing, and reporting of non-interventional studies that utilise real-world data for safety assessment of medicines. EMA/CHMP/ICH/155061/2024. Amsterdam (NL): EMA; 2025.

15. Kirby JC, Speltz P, Rasmussen LV, Basford M, Gottesman O, Peissig PL, et al. PheKB: a catalog and workflow for creating electronic phenotype algorithms for electronic health records. J Am Med Inform Assoc. 2016;23(6):1046-1052.

16. Enewold L, Parsons H, Zhao L, Bott D, Rivera DR, Barrett MJ, et al. Updated overview of the SEER–Medicare data: enhanced content and applications. J Natl Cancer Inst Monogr. 2020;2020(55):3-13. doi:10.1093/jncimonographs/lgz029.

17. Jernberg T, Attebring MF, Hambraeus K, Ivert T, James S, Jeppsson A, et al. The Swedish Web-system for enhancement and development of evidence-based care in heart disease evaluated according to recommended therapies (SWEDEHEART). Heart. 2010;96(20):1617-1621. doi:10.1136/hrt.2010.198804.

18. Perez MV, Mahaffey KW, Hedlin H, Rumsfeld JS, Garcia A, Ferris T, et al. Large-Scale Assessment of a Smartwatch to Identify Atrial Fibrillation. N Engl J Med. 2019 Nov 14;381(20):1909-17. doi: 10.1056/NEJMoa1901183.

19. Hripcsak G, et al. Characterizing treatment pathways at scale using the OHDSI network. Proc Natl Acad Sci USA. 2016;113(27):7329–7336.

20. EU Commission. EHDEN Project Deliverable D6.1: Data Processing Infrastructure. 2021.

21. Arlett P, Kjaer J, Broich K, et al. Real-world evidence in EU medicines regulation: enabling use and establishing value. Clin Pharmacol Ther. 2022;111(1):21-23.

22. Medical Data Vision Co., Ltd. MDV Database Specifications. 2023.

23. Hripcsak G, Albers DJ. Next-generation phenotyping of electronic health records. J Am Med Inform Assoc. 2013;20(1):117-121. doi:10.1136/amiajnl-2012-001145.

24. Hughes RA, Heron J, Sterne JAC, Tilling K. Accounting for missing data in statistical analyses: multiple imputation is not always the answer. Int J Epidemiol. 2019;48(4):1294-1304. doi:10.1093/ije/dyz032.

25. Austin PC. An introduction to propensity score methods for reducing the effects of confounding in observational studies. Multivariate Behav Res. 2011;46(3):399–424.

26. Wang SV, et al. Use of high-dimensional propensity scores in observational pharmacoepidemiology. Am J Epidemiol. 2022;191(10):1735–1743.

27. Robins JM, Hernán MA, Brumback B. Marginal structural models and causal inference in epidemiology. Epidemiology. 2000;11(5):550–560.

28. Patone M, Mei XW, Handunnetthi L, Dixon S, Zaccardi F, Shankar-Hari M, et al. Risk of myocarditis after COVID-19 vaccination in England. Circulation. 2022;146(20):1537-1547. doi:10.1161/CIRCULATIONAHA.122.060785.

29. Klein NP, Lewis N, Goddard K, Fireman B, Zerbo O, Hanson KE, et al. Surveillance for adverse events after COVID-19 mRNA vaccination. JAMA. 2021;326(14):1390-1399. doi:10.1001/jama.2021.15072.

30. Lipsitch M, Tchetgen Tchetgen E, Cohen T. Negative controls: a tool for detecting confounding and bias in observational studies. Epidemiology. 2010;21(3):383–388.

31. Schuemie MJ, Hripcsak G, Ryan PB, Madigan D. Robust empirical calibration of p-values using observational data. Stat Med. 2016;35(22):3883-3888.

32. VanderWeele TJ, Ding P. Sensitivity analysis in observational research: introducing the E-value. Ann Intern Med. 2017;167(4):268–274.

33. Westreich D, Edwards JK, Lesko CR, Stuart EA, Cole SR. Transportability of trial results using inverse odds of sampling weights. Am J Epidemiol. 2017;186(8):1010-1014.

34. FDA. Biologics License Application for Aducanumab (Aduhelm). Statistical Review. 2021.

35. von Elm E, Altman DG, Egger M, Pocock SJ, Gøtzsche PC, Vandenbroucke JP; STROBE Initiative. The Strengthening the Reporting of Observational Studies in Epidemiology (STROBE) statement: guidelines for reporting observational studies. Lancet. 2007;370(9596):1453-1457.

36. Benchimol EI, et al. The REporting of studies Conducted using Observational Routinely-collected health Data (RECORD) statement. PLoS Med. 2015;12(10):e1001885.

37. Langan SM, Schmidt SAJ, Wing K, Ehrenstein V, Nicholls SG, Filion KB, et al. The Reporting of Studies Conducted Using Observational Routinely-Collected Health Data (RECORD) for pharmacoepidemiology (RECORD-PE) statement. BMJ. 2018;363:k3532.

# Chapter 6. Real-World Study Designs

Observational studies constitute the backbone of real-world evidence (RWE) generation. Unlike randomized controlled trials (RCTs), which impose strict experimental control, observational studies capture data as they naturally occur in routine clinical practice, registries, administrative databases, and patient-generated sources. Their strength lies in external validity - i.e., generalizability to heterogeneous populations - and in the feasibility of addressing questions where randomization is *irrelevant, impractical, unethical*, or simply *unaffordable*. However, this freedom from experimental control introduces systematic differences between exposure groups - confounding - that must be anticipated, measured, and mitigated through rigorous design and analysis.

A unifying principle for designing robust observational RWE studies is *target trial emulation*: before extracting data or specifying models, investigators should articulate the randomized controlled trial they would ideally conduct to answer their question - including eligibility criteria, treatment strategies, outcome definitions, and follow-up duration - and then emulate that design as faithfully as possible using real-world data. This approach reduces self-inflicted biases (e.g., immortal time) and clarifies where data limitations may compromise validity. Operationally, RWE studies benefit from a three-layer workflow:

- **Design layer** that specifies cohort assembly and temporal anchors
- **Measurement layer** that transforms raw data streams into valid exposure, outcome, and confounder variables; and
- **Analysis layer** that estimates causal effects while accounting for data-generating mechanisms [1].

This structured progression ensures that analytical sophistication serves, rather than obscures, the underlying causal question.

This chapter details the four principal observational study designs used in RWE: cohort, case–control, cross-sectional, and nested designs. The emphasis remains on design-level rigor - because no amount of statistical adjustment can fully compensate for a poorly conceived study.

# 6.1. Cohort Studies

## 6.1.1. Definition and Core Structure

A cohort study follows a defined group of individuals over time, classifying them at baseline by exposure status (e.g., drug use, surgical intervention, lifestyle factor) and tracking incident outcomes. The temporal sequence - exposure before outcome - is inherent to the design, which affords a natural framework for causal inference when confounding is adequately controlled [2]. Figure 6.1 shows a cohort study flow.

Cohorts may be **prospective** (follow-up initiated after exposure ascertainment using primary data collection) or **retrospective** (exposure and outcome data extracted from pre-existing secondary data, with follow-up occurring in calendar past time). In RWE, the latter is far more common, especially when leveraging electronic health records (EHRs), claims databases, or existing disease registries.

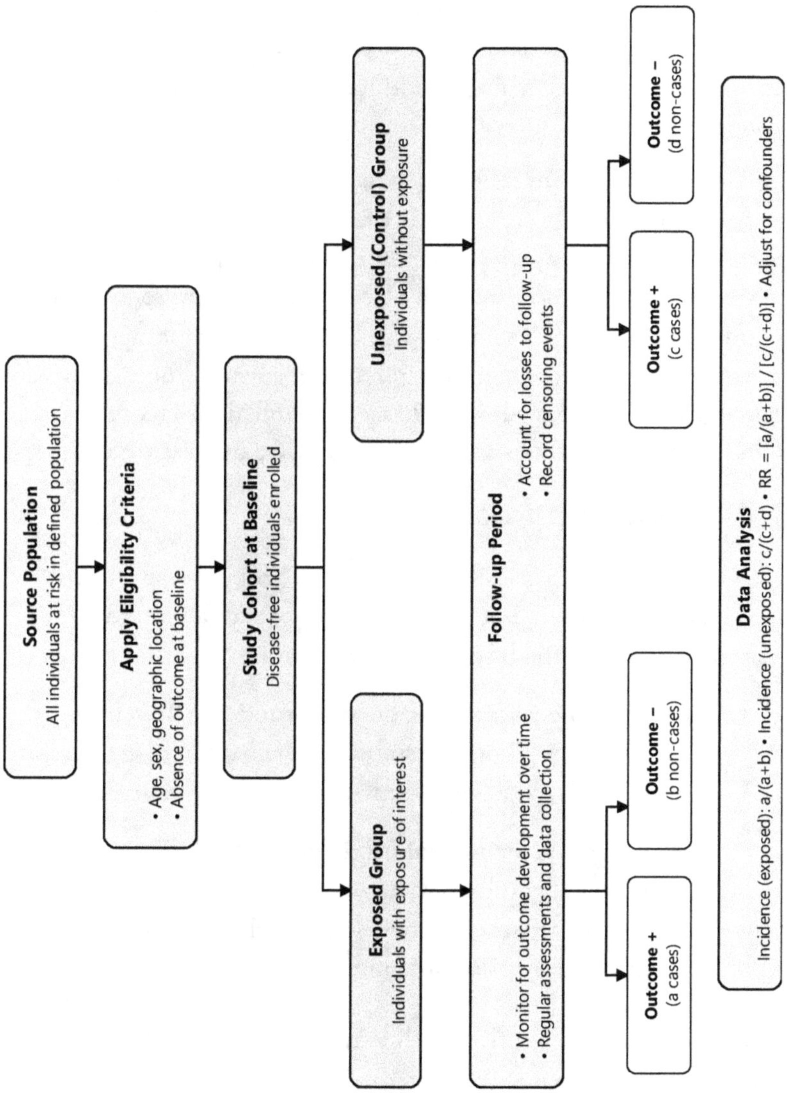


**Figure 6.1. Cohort Study Flow**

## 6.1.2. Key Design Considerations

Designing a robust cohort study in the real-world setting begins well before statistical analysis - with deliberate, transparent decisions about how the cohort is assembled, how exposure and outcomes are defined, how follow-up is managed, and how potential sources of bias are anticipated.

Unlike randomized trials, where allocation and protocol adherence are enforced, observational cohorts rely on *pre-existing data structures* and *clinical practice patterns*; therefore, every eligibility criterion, temporal rule, and validation step must be codified a priori to minimize design-induced distortion. Table 6.1 synthesizes key methodological checkpoints that have proven critical in recent regulatory submissions and methodological guidance, with specific recommendations tailored to common RWE data sources such as claims, EHRs, and disease registries.

## 6.1.3. Analytical Approaches

Time-to-event analysis is standard. Cox proportional hazards models remain widely used, but violation of proportional hazards (e.g., time-varying treatment effects) warrants alternatives:

- **Flexible parametric survival models (Royston–Parmar)** [6] - allow smooth baseline hazard estimation and can incorporate time-dependent covariates.
- **Marginal structural models (MSMs)** with inverse probability of treatment weighting (IPTW) - especially when exposure is time-varying and confounding is affected by prior outcomes [7].

A final analytical consideration is the choice of causal *estimand*. The *on-treatment* effect estimates the outcome difference while patients remain on the index therapy, censoring at discontinuation; it is clinically intuitive but vulnerable to informative censoring if discontinuation correlates with early outcomes.

**Table 6.1. Key Considerations in Designing a Cohort Study**

| Consideration | Guidance for RWE Context |
|---|---|
| **Cohort definition** | Define eligibility criteria using observable variables (e.g., ICD-10 codes, prescription fills, laboratory thresholds). Avoid criteria requiring non structured data unless a validated NLP algorithm is available. |
| **Exposure ascertainment** | Use a new-user design whenever possible: restrict to patients initiating the exposure at study entry to minimize immortal time bias [3]. When possible employ un active comparator (e.g. another drug in the same class)) to reduce confounding by indication. Clarify exposure windows (e.g., ≥2 consecutive fills for chronic therapy) and define a cohort entry date as the primary temporal anchor, with pre-specified covariate assessment, washout and follow-up windows. |
| **Follow-up window** | Align with regulatory expectations: FDA often expects ≥1 year of post-exposure observation for safety endpoints; EMA may accept shorter windows if justified by disease natural history (e.g., acute infection). |
| **Outcome definition** | Prefer validated algorithms (e.g., PPV ≥80% for myocardial infarction) [4]; OHDSI's phenotype library [5]). Document positive predictive value (PPV) and sensitivity where available. |
| **Loss to follow-up** | In claims data, administrative censoring (e.g., insurance disenrollment) is common; treat as informative censoring and apply inverse probability weighting or sensitivity analyses. |
| **Temporal window specification** | Define pre-exposure covariate assessment windows (to avoid adjusting for causal intermediates), outcome washout periods (to ensure incident events), and biologically plausible effect windows for follow-up. Document grace periods for exposure continuity and justify their duration based on pharmacokinetics and disease natural history [1]. |

The *as-started* effect (analogous to *intention-to-treat*) follows patients regardless of subsequent treatment changes, avoiding censoring bias but potentially diluting effects through exposure misclassification over time. When treatment strategies are complex (e.g., dose titration, switching), marginal structural models or g-estimation may be required to address time-varying confounding [7]. Pre-specifying the target estimand - and justifying its clinical relevance - is essential for transparent interpretation.

### 6.1.4. Illustrative Example: Post-Marketing Safety Surveillance Using a New-User, Active-Comparator Cohort Design

A landmark post-marketing safety study conducted by FDA investigators, illustrates how a new-user, active-comparator cohort design can generate credible real-world evidence that both corroborates and extends RCT findings [8].

The study assembled propensity score–matched cohorts of elderly Medicare patients initiating dabigatran or warfarin for nonvalvular atrial fibrillation between 2010 and 2012, yielding 134,414 patients and 37,587 person-years of follow-up. Warfarin served as the active comparator - the established therapeutic alternative for the same indication - directly addressing confounding by indication in a way a placebo or non-user comparator could not.

Propensity score matching balanced baseline characteristics across cohorts, producing hazard ratios for dabigatran vs. warfarin of: ischemic stroke 0.80 (95% CI 0.67–0.96), acute myocardial infarction 0.92 (95% CI 0.78-1.08), intracranial haemorrhage 0.34 (95% CI 0.26–0.46), major gastrointestinal bleeding 1.28 (95% CI 1.14–1.44), and all-cause mortality 0.86 (95% CI 0.77–0.96). This differentiated outcome profile - benefit on stroke and intracranial bleeding but harm on gastrointestinal bleeding - illustrates why pre-specifying a comprehensive, multi-outcome set is essential. Dose-stratified analyses further revealed that the 150 mg dose drove most of the divergent effects, adding clinically actionable nuance unavailable from the pivotal RE-LY trial [9].

This study exemplifies the core principles of rigorous pharmacoepidemiological cohort research: new-user design, active comparator, propensity score matching with transparent balance diagnostics, pre-specified multiple outcomes, and dose-stratified sensitivity analyses.

## 6.2. Case–Control Studies

Case–control studies begin with the identification of individuals who have experienced the outcome of interest (cases) and a comparable set who have not (controls). Researchers then retrospectively assess exposure history. Efficiency is the hallmark: when outcomes are rare (e.g., drug-induced agranulocytosis), a case–control design can achieve high statistical power with far fewer subjects than a cohort study [2].

Two primary variants exist in RWE:

- **Traditional (incident) case–control**: Cases are newly diagnosed; controls are sampled from the same source population at risk.  show a traditional case-control study flow. Figure 6.2 shows a traditional case-control study flow.
- **Case–crossover:** Each case serves as his/her own control, comparing exposure during a hazard period (e.g., 7 days before event) with exposure during a control period (e.g., 30 days before) [10]. Figure 6.3 shows a case-cross over study flow.

### 6.2.1. Matching and Control Selection

Control selection profoundly influences bias. Three widely used strategies exist:

- **Risk-set sampling (incidence density sampling)**: For each case, select controls from the population *at risk* at the time of case occurrence. This preserves the underlying person-time structure and yields odds ratios approximating incidence rate ratios [11].
- **Case–control within a cohort (nested case–control)**: Controls sampled from the same cohort that generated cases - discussed later.
- **Disease-free prevalent sampling**: Controls drawn irrespective of time, which can introduce *prevalence bias* if exposure prevalence changes over calendar time.

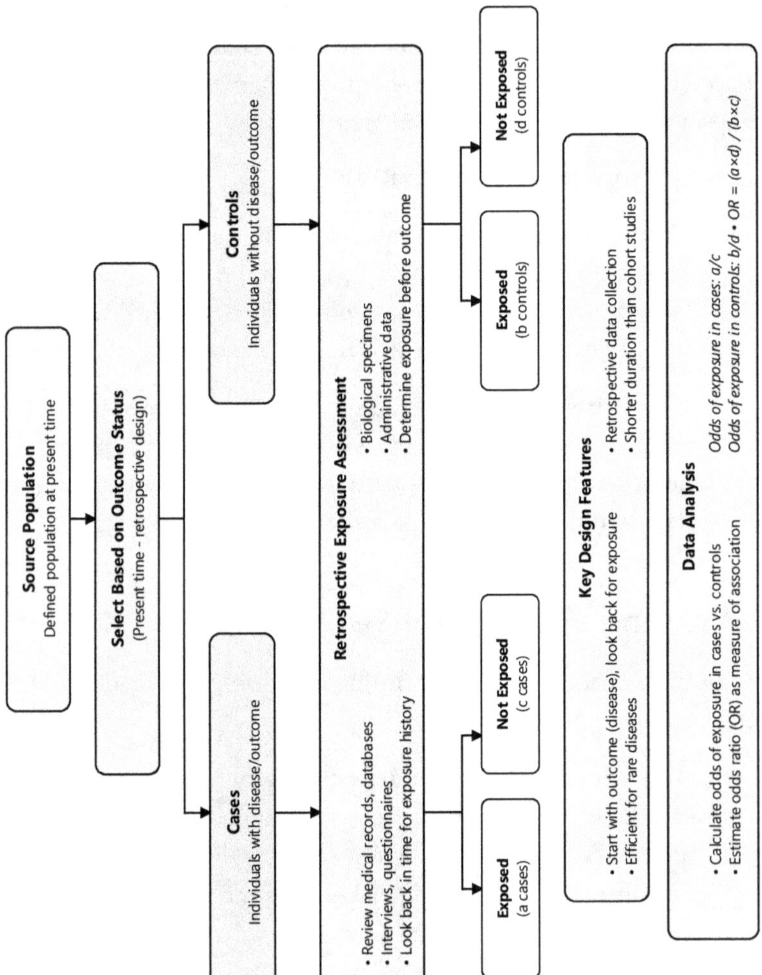


**Figure 6.2. Traditional (incident) Case–Control Study Flow**

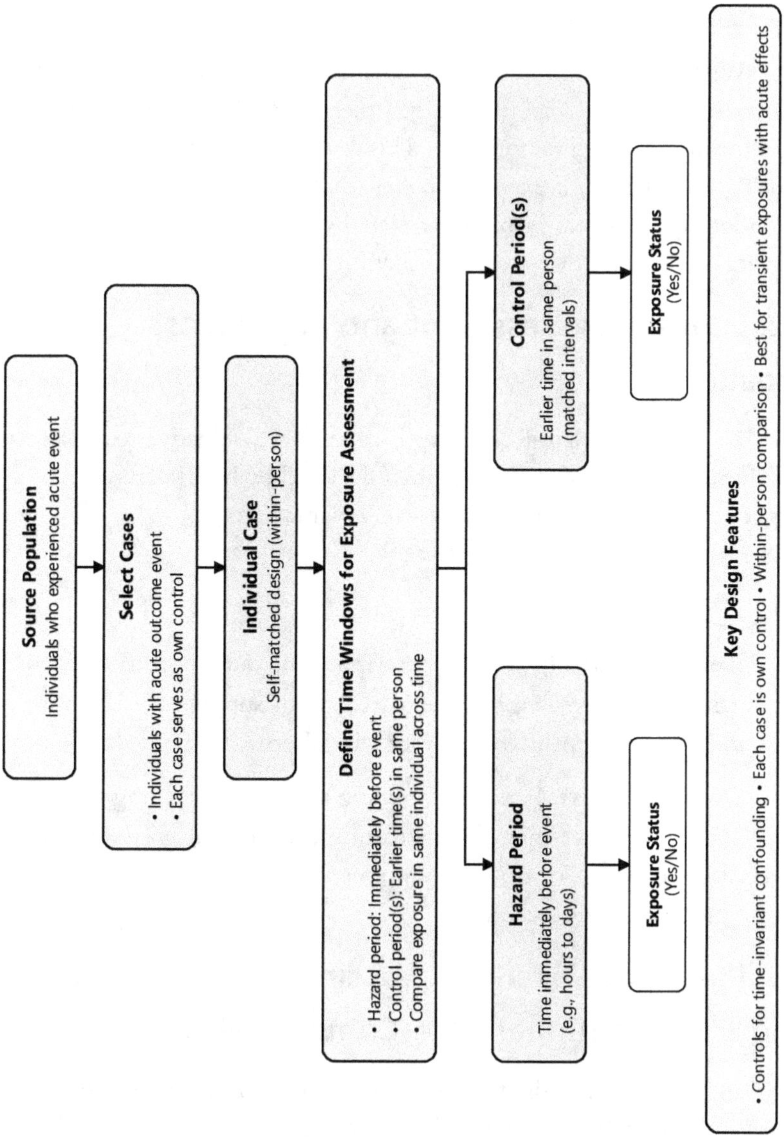


**Figure 6.3. Case–Crossover Study Flow**

When matching, avoid *overmatching* on variables that lie on the causal pathway (e.g., matching on hospitalization status when studying post-discharge medication adherence). Matching variables must be pre-specified and justified a priori.

When residual confounding remains a concern despite careful matching, high-dimensional proxy adjustment (hdPS) can strengthen control for unmeasured factors [12]. This approach algorithmically screens thousands of pre-exposure codes (diagnoses, procedures, drug fills) to identify empirical proxies correlated with latent confounders (e.g., healthcare utilization intensity as a proxy for frailty).

### 6.2.2. Exposure Assessment and Recall Bias Mitigation

In secondary data RWE, exposure data are objective (e.g., prescription fills, lab orders) rather than declared by healthcare professionals, eliminating recall bias - an advantage over questionnaire-based epidemiology.

However, misclassification remains:

**Temporal ambiguity**: A prescription fill date may not reflect actual ingestion. Use *exposure windows* (e.g., days of supply + 7-day grace period) and conduct sensitivity analyses with alternative windows.

**Database gaps**: Patients switching insurers or moving to fee-for-service may have incomplete histories. Implement *washout periods* (e.g., require ≥180 days of prior continuous enrollment) to ensure exposure ascertainment reliability.

### 6.2.3. Illustrative Example: Vaccine Safety Surveillance Using a Multinational Case-Control Design

A European multinational case-control study assessed the association between the adjuvanted pandemic influenza A (H1N1) 2009 vaccine and Guillain-Barré syndrome (GBS) across five European countries [13]. Neurologist-confirmed GBS cases - classified using the Brighton Collaboration case definition - were matched to controls on age, sex, index date, and country. It internationally validated, adjudicated case definition ensured consistent outcome ascertainment across countries, preventing differential misclassification.

After conditional logistic regression adjusting for antecedent respiratory infection and prior seasonal vaccination, pandemic vaccine was not associated with increased GBS risk (adjusted OR 1.0, 95% CI 0.3–2.7). Critically, the precision of the estimate allowed quantification of an upper boundary of three excess GBS cases per million vaccinated individuals - a directly actionable finding for regulators. The study demonstrates the core strengths of a well-executed case-control design: a rare outcome making cohort approaches infeasible; standardized adjudicated case ascertainment; population-based control sampling; and multinational pooling to achieve adequate power under time pressure.

## 6.3. Cross-Sectional Studies

Cross-sectional studies collect exposure and outcome data simultaneously at a single time point. They are primarily descriptive- ideal for estimating disease prevalence, health service utilization patterns, or associations where temporality is less critical (e.g., comorbidity clustering). Unlike cohort or case-control designs, cross-sectional studies cannot establish incidence or directionality, limiting causal inference [2]. shows the data snapshot of a cross-sectional study. In RWE, cross-sectional analyses often serve as *baseline characterizations* for longitudinal studies or as rapid situation assessments (e.g., pandemic surveillance).

### 6.3.1. Design Strengths and Pitfalls

Cross-sectional studies offer distinct methodological trade-offs: their efficiency and immediacy are counterbalanced by inherent limitations in causal inference and susceptibility to specific biases. Understanding these dualities is essential when deciding whether a cross-sectional design is fit for purpose - and when interpreting its findings in regulatory or clinical contexts.

**Table 6.2. Strengths and Pitfalls of Cross-Sectional Studies**

| Strength | Pitfall |
|---|---|
| Rapid, low-cost assessment of prevalence and multimorbidity patterns | Inability to infer causality (reverse causation, e.g., depression may be a consequence - not cause - of chronic pain) |
| Enables hypothesis generation for longitudinal studies | Susceptible to selection bias if data capture varies by outcome status (e.g., sicker patients have more frequent encounters, inflating exposure detection) |
| Compatible with national health surveys and registry snapshots | Prevalence estimates may be distorted by differential survival (Neyman bias) |

## 6.3.2. Analytical Approaches

Because both exposure and outcome are binary or categorical, logistic regression is commonly used, but interpretation shifts to *prevalence odds ratios* (PORs) rather than risk or rate ratios. When the outcome is common (>10% prevalence), PORs overstate the prevalence ratio (PR); use log-binomial or robust Poisson regression to estimate PRs directly [14, 15].

Weighting is frequently required to align the sample with the target population (e.g., post-stratification by age, sex, region using census data), especially when using convenience samples (e.g., single-center EHR extracts).

## 6.3.3. Illustrative Example: Prevalence of Potentially Inappropriate Medications in French Nursing Homes

A 2023 cross-sectional study used the French National Health Data System (SNDS) to estimate the prevalence of potentially inappropriate medications (PIMs) among 274,971 nursing home residents (NHRs) aged ≥75 years across France over a three-month period in 2019 [16].

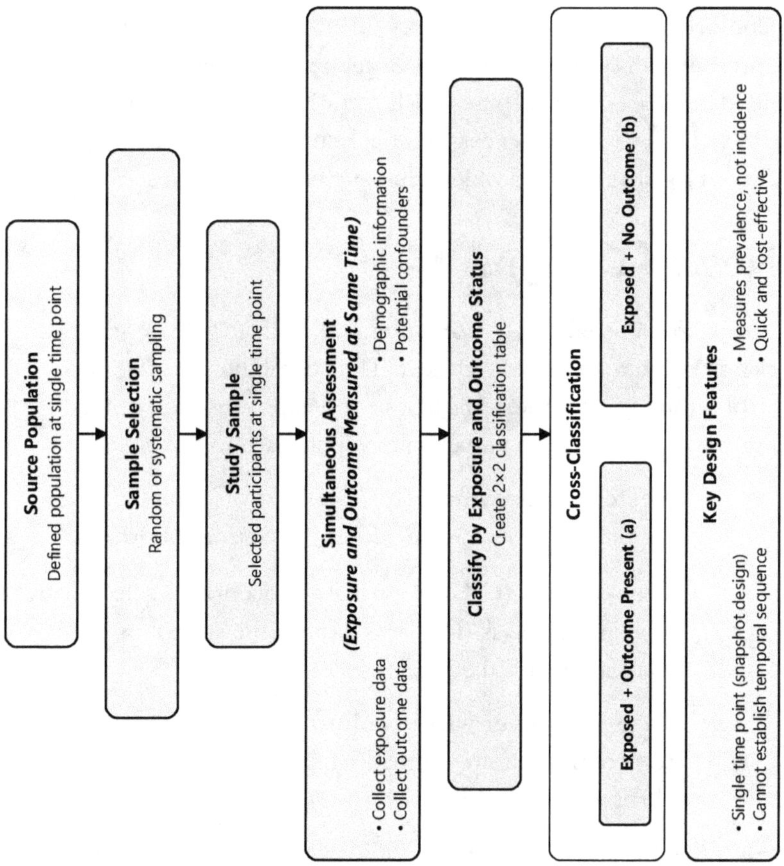


**Figure 6.4. Cross-Sectional Design Snapshot**

Because the crude PIM prevalence exceeded 10%, multivariable robust Poisson regression was applied to estimate adjusted prevalence ratios (aPRs) directly - a methodological choice that avoids the well-known overestimation of effect size produced by odds ratios under common outcomes. The study found that 54% of NHRs received at least one PIM, compared with 29% of community-dwelling older adults, with NHRs remaining 33% more likely to receive a PIM after adjustment for age, sex, comorbidities, and polypharmacy (aPR = 1.33; 95% CI 1.33–1.34); co-prescription of three or more central nervous system-active drugs (aPR = 1.94), benzodiazepines (aPR = 1.43), and anticholinergic agents (aPR = 1.29) drove the excess, highlighting the particular vulnerability of institutionalized older adults to suboptimal prescribing.

## 6.4. Nested Designs

Nested designs embed a more intensive study (e.g., case–control or case–cohort) within an existing cohort. They combine the *efficiency* of case–control sampling with the *temporal rigor* and exposure clarity of a cohort framework. Three main variants are widely used in RWE:

1. **Nested case–control (NCC)**: Controls sampled from the risk set of each case within the parent cohort.
2. **Case–cohort (C-C)**: A random subcohort is selected at baseline; all cases (inside or outside the subcohort) are compared with the subcohort.
3. **Case–crossover within cohort**: Each case's hazard and control periods are defined relative to the cohort's observation window.

All three preserve the internal validity advantages of the cohort while reducing data collection burden - crucial when high-dimensional covariates (e.g., genomics, imaging) are costly to obtain.

### 6.4.1. Statistical Analysis

- **NCC:** Conditional logistic regression, with stratification by risk set (matched set) inherently adjusts for matching variables.

- **C-C**: Weighted Cox regression (Prentice weights) or pseudolikelihood approaches; software packages (e.g., *survival* in R) implement these efficiently [17].
- **Variance estimation:** Standard errors must reflect the sampling design; bootstrapping across risk sets is recommended for small numbers of cases.

### 6.4.2. Efficiency Gains

Simulation studies show that generally a 1:4 NCC design achieves ≥90% of the statistical power of a full cohort analysis while reducing data abstraction by about >75% [18]. This is especially valuable when outcomes are rare (e.g., vaccine-associated thrombosis with thrombocytopenia syndrome, incidence ~1 per 100 000 doses).

An additional efficiency advantage of the case-cohort design is that the randomly selected sub-cohort can be reused to study multiple outcomes without re-sampling, making it particularly valuable for *post-authorization safety studies* where several endpoints (e.g., cardiovascular events, renal outcomes, hypoglycemia) may be evaluated from the same source population [1].

### 6.4.3. Illustrative Example: Opioid Use and Dementia Risk

A 2024 nationwide nested case–control study assessed the association between cumulative noncancer opioid use and incident all-cause dementia within a Danish population-based cohort of 1,872,854 individuals followed from 2000 through 2020 [19]. Among these, 93,638 (5.0%) developed dementia during follow-up and were each incidence-density matched by age and sex to five dementia-free controls, yielding 468,190 controls drawn from the same dynamic risk set. Exposure was defined as cumulative opioid fills expressed in total standardized doses (TSDs), with a five-year lag-time window applied to mitigate reverse causation - a methodological safeguard essential when the outcome may itself precipitate the exposure. Conditional logistic regression found no significant association below 90 TSDs, but demonstrated a clear dose-response gradient at higher levels: adjusted incidence rate ratios were 1.28

(95% CI 1.16–1.41), 1.44 (95% CI 1.28–1.62), and 1.58 (95% CI 1.43–1.75) for the 91–200, 201–500, and >500 TSD categories respectively, consistent across both weak and strong opioid subgroups.

## 6.5. Comparative Summary and Selection Guidance

Choosing the optimal observational design hinges on three factors: (1) the research question (incidence vs. prevalence vs. rare event), (2) data availability (longitudinal depth, granularity), and (3) resource constraints (cost of chart review, molecular testing). Table 6.2 synthesizes core attributes.

## 6.6. Conclusion

In summary, observational study designs - cohort, case–control, cross-sectional, and nested variants - provide complementary tools for generating real-world evidence, each with distinct temporal logic, efficiency profiles, and vulnerability to bias. Their appropriate selection, meticulous protocolization, and transparent reporting are not merely technical choices but foundational determinants of evidentiary credibility. As regulators increasingly accept RWE to support label expansions, safety monitoring, and comparative effectiveness assessments [24, 25], mastery of these designs - grounded in target trial emulation, rigorous measurement, transparent reporting, and thoughtful sensitivity analyses - becomes indispensable for researchers, sponsors, and health authorities alike.

**Table 6.2. Comparative Attributes of Observational Designs in RWE**

| Design | Temporal Direction | Typical Outcome Frequency | Sample Size Efficiency | Key Bias Threats | Regulatory Acceptance Examples |
|---|---|---|---|---|---|
| **Cohort (prospective/ retrospective)** | Exposure → Outcome | Any (preferred for common outcomes) | Moderate–Low (requires full cohort) | Confounding, immortal time bias | FDA's RWE Framework (2023) accepts new-user cohort for label expansions [20] |
| **Case–Control (incident)** | Outcome ← Exposure | Rare (≤5%) | High | Selection bias, recall bias (mitigated in RWE) | EMA's Guideline on observational studies endorses for safety signal confirmation [21] |
| **Cross-Sectional** | Simultaneous | Prevalence estimation | Very High | Reverse causation, survival bias | WHO's STEPwise approach uses cross-sectional surveys for NCD monitoring [22] |
| **Nested Case–Control** | Exposure → Outcome (within cohort) | Rare | Very High | Same as cohort, plus sampling variability | FDA's Sentinel Initiative employs NCC for rapid safety assessments [23] |
| **Case–Cohort** | Exposure → Outcome (partial cohort) | Any | High | Subcohort selection bias (if not random) | Used in the Canadian AVID study for vaccine effectiveness [24] |

Note: "Regulatory Acceptance Examples" reflect formal guidance or precedent decisions, not exhaustive lists.

## References

1. Schneeweiss S, Patorno E. Conducting real-world evidence studies on the clinical outcomes of diabetes treatments. Endocr Rev. 2021;42(5):658-690.

2. Lash TL, VanderWeele TJ, Haneuse S, Rothman KJ. Modern Epidemiology. 4th ed. Wolters Kluwer; 2021.

3. Suissa S. Immortal time bias in pharmacoepidemiology. Am J Epidemiol. 2008 Feb 15;167(4):492-9. doi: 10.1093/aje/kwm324.

4. Kawai AT, et al. Validity of a high-specificity algorithm for acute myocardial infarction in US administrative claims. Pharmacoepidemiol Drug Saf. 2020;29(3):283-292.

5. Observational Health Data Sciences and Informatics (OHDSI). Phenotype Library. https://github.com/ohdsi/PhenotypeLibrary. Accessed 2025.

6. Royston P, Parmar MK. Flexible parametric proportional-hazards and proportional-odds models for censored survival data. Stat Med. 2002;21(6):895-913. doi:10.1002/sim.1203

7. Robins JM, et al. Marginal structural models and causal inference in epidemiology. Epidemiology. 2000;11(5):550-560.

8. Graham DJ, Reichman ME, Wernecke M, Zhang R, Southworth MR, Levenson M, et al. Cardiovascular, bleeding, and mortality risks in elderly Medicare patients treated with dabigatran or warfarin for nonvalvular atrial fibrillation. Circulation. 2015;131(2):157–164. doi:10.1161/CIRCULATIONAHA.114.012061

9. Connolly SJ, Ezekowitz MD, Yusuf S, Eikelboom J, Oldgren J, Parekh A, et al.; RE-LY Steering Committee and Investigators. Dabigatran versus warfarin in patients with atrial fibrillation. N Engl J Med. 2009;361(12):1139–1151. doi:10.1056/NEJMoa0905561

10. Maclure M. The case-crossover design: a method for studying transient effects on the risk of acute events. Am J Epidemiol. 1991;133(2):144-153.

11. Rothman KJ, Huybrechts KF, Murray EJ. Epidemiology: An Introduction. 3rd ed. New York: Oxford University Press; 2024.

12. Schneeweiss S, Rassen JA, Glynn RJ, Avorn J, Mogun H, Brookhart MA. High-dimensional propensity score adjustment in studies of treatment effects using health care claims data. Epidemiology. 2009;20(4):512–522. doi:10.1097/EDE.0b013e3181a663cc. PMID: 19487948

13. Dieleman J, Romio S, Johansen K, Weibel D, Bonhoeffer J, Sturkenboom M; VAESCO-GBS Case-Control Study Group. Guillain-Barré syndrome and adjuvanted pandemic influenza A (H1N1) 2009 vaccine: multinational case-control study in Europe. BMJ. 2011;343:d3908. doi:10.1136/bmj.d3908. PMID: 21750072

14. Zou G. A modified Poisson regression approach to prospective studies with binary data. Am J Epidemiol. 2004;159(7):702–706.

15. Barros AJ, Hirakata VN. Alternatives for logistic regression in cross-sectional studies: an empirical comparison of models that directly estimate the prevalence ratio. BMC Med Res Methodol. 2003;3:21.

16. Drusch S, Le Tri T, Ankri J, Michelon H, Zureik M, Herr M. Potentially inappropriate medications in nursing homes and the community older adults using the French health insurance databases. Pharmacoepidemiol Drug Saf. 2023;32(4):475–485. doi:10.1002/pds.5575.

17. Prentice RL. A case-cohort design for epidemiologic cohort studies and disease prevention trials. Biometrika. 1986;73(1):1-11.

18. Langholz B, Thomas DC. Nested case-control and case-cohort methods of sampling from a cohort: a critical comparison. Am J Epidemiol. 1990;131(1):169–176.

19. Pourhadi N, Janbek J, Gasse C, Laursen TM, Waldemar G, Jensen-Dahm C. Opioids and dementia in the Danish population. JAMA Netw Open. 2024;7(11):e2445904. doi:10.1001/jamanetworkopen.2024.45904 21.

20. US Food and Drug Administration. Considerations for the Use of Real-World Data and Real-World Evidence to Support Regulatory

Decision-Making for Drug and Biological Products. Guidance for Industry; August 2024.

21. European Medicines Agency. Guideline on good pharmacovigilance practices (GVP) Module VIII – Post-authorisation safety studies. Rev. 2 (2022).

22. World Health Organization. STEPwise approach to surveillance (STEPS). 2023 update.

23. Curtis LH, et al. The FDA's Sentinel Initiative: expanding real-world evidence for regulatory decision-making. Clin Pharmacol Ther. 2022;111(3):543-551.

24. Kwong JC, et al. The AVID study: a case–cohort design to evaluate influenza vaccine effectiveness in Canada. Vaccine. 2021;39(45):6612-6620.

25. Arlett P, et al. Real-world evidence in EU medicines regulation: enabling use and establishing value through Darwin EU. Front Pharmacol. 2024;15:1350438.

# Chapter 7. Understanding Bias and Confounding

Real-world evidence (RWE) studies are indispensable for informing clinical decision-making, regulatory decisions, health policy, and value-based healthcare - yet their credibility hinges critically on how well investigators anticipate, assess, and mitigate bias and confounding. Unlike randomized controlled trials (RCTs), where randomization and blinding serve as structural safeguards, observational studies rely on design, measurement, and analytical ingenuity to approximate causal inference. Bias and confounding are not mere technical footnotes: they are the principal threats to internal validity in RWE. A well-crafted RWE study does not eliminate all bias - this is rarely possible - but rather renders its influence transparent, quantifiable, and, where feasible, minimized.

This chapter provides a systematic exploration of bias and confounding in RWE, distinguishing their origins, manifestations, and interdependence, and detailing contemporary strategies for their mitigation. Emphasis is placed on practical implementation informed by recent methodological guidance from the U.S. Food and Drug Administration (FDA), the European Medicines Agency (EMA), the

International Council for Harmonization (ICH), and the International Society for Pharmacoeconomics and Outcomes Research (ISPOR).

## 7.1. Types of Bias

Bias in RWE refers to any **systematic deviation** from the truth in the estimation of an association or effect, arising from flaws in study design, data collection, analysis, or interpretation. Biases are not random errors; they consistently skew results in a particular direction and, if unaddressed, may lead to erroneous conclusions about effectiveness, safety, or value. Though numerous taxonomies exist, we organize bias in RWE into four broad, overlapping categories: **selection bias**, **information (measurement) bias**, **time-related bias**, and **analysis bias**. Each arises from distinct mechanisms and requires tailored mitigation strategies.

### 7.1.1. Selection Bias

Selection bias occurs when the process of enrolling or retaining participants systematically differs between exposure or outcome groups, leading to a non-representative sample. In RWE, this is especially problematic given the frequent reliance on healthcare databases, registries, or electronic health records (EHRs) where eligibility and inclusion are driven by clinical, administrative, or technical factors - not just a scientific protocol.

A canonical example is **immortal time bias**, a subset of selection bias in which a period of follow-up time is misclassified, often because the exposed cohort must survive long enough to receive the exposure. For instance, in a study evaluating the effect of statin initiation on mortality after myocardial infarction (MI), if time from MI to first statin prescription is excluded from the "exposed" person-time and instead misattributed to the "unexposed" group, the unexposed group gains artificially elevated risk - yielding an artificial protective effect for statins [1]. Similar distortions arise in studies of cancer therapies where treatment eligibility requires surviving a minimum period post-diagnosis - creating a "survivor" selection effect [2]. Figure 7.1 depicts the flow of immortal time bias.

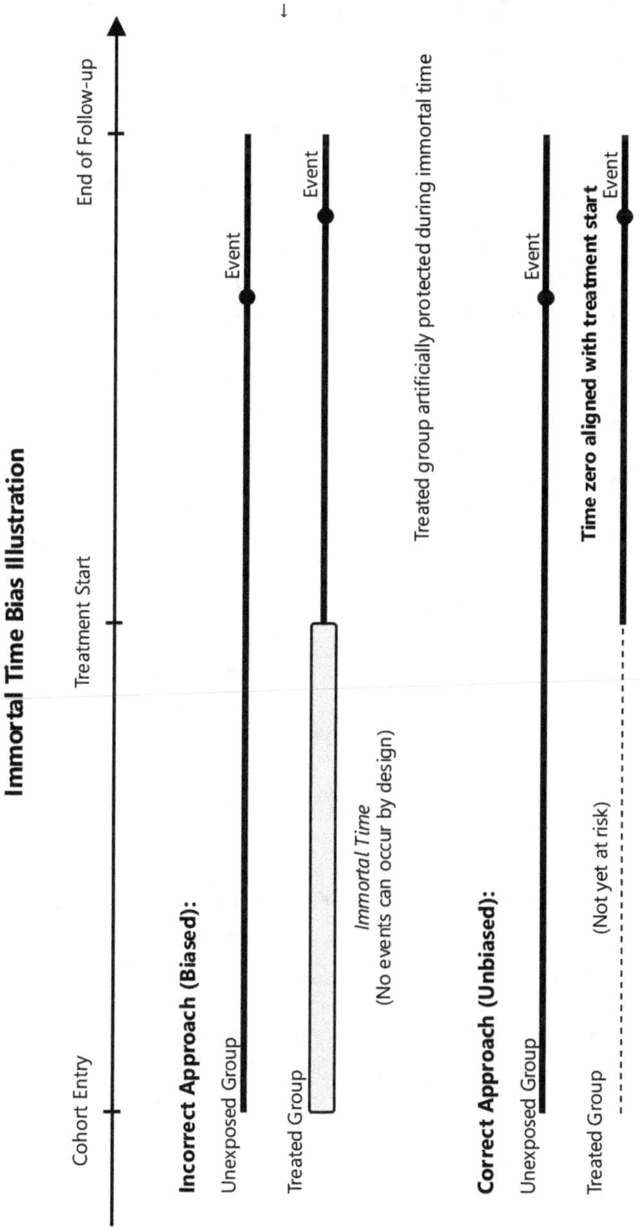


**Figure 7.1. Immortal Time Bias**

**Table 7.1. Common Types of Selection Bias in RWE**

| Type of Bias | Mechanism | Example |
|---|---|---|
| **Immortal time bias** | Misclassification of person-time before exposure | Statin study where time from MI to first prescription is assigned to unexposed group [1] |
| **Prevalent user bias** | Inclusion of long-term users at baseline | Evaluation of long-acting bronchodilators in COPD including patients already on therapy for >6 months [3] |
| **Healthy user bias** | Exposure linked to health-conscious behaviors | Observational studies of vitamin D supplementation showing reduced cardiovascular risk, confounded by lifestyle factors [4] |
| **Loss-to-follow-up bias** | Differential attrition by exposure or outcome status | EHR-based study where patients discontinuing a biologic (due to adverse events) exit care systems and become unobservable [5] |
| **Administrative selection bias** | Eligibility determined by insurance or coding rules | Medicare claims study excluding dual-eligible patients, limiting generalizability to socioeconomically vulnerable populations [6] |

Table 7.1 provides common types of selection bias. Other forms include:

- **Prevalent user bias**: when analyses include individuals already using a therapy at study entry, conflating long-term survivors (who are inherently lower risk) with incident users.
- **Channeling bias**: where clinicians preferentially prescribe certain treatments to patients with specific prognostic profiles (e.g., reserving newer anticoagulants for younger, healthier patients), generating non-random exposure allocation.
- **Database entry bias**: in registries or claims databases, differential coding practices or data capture (e.g., more thorough comorbidity documentation in sicker patients) can distort exposure - outcome associations.

## 7.1.2. Information (Measurement) Bias

Information bias arises when data on exposure, outcome, covariates, or follow-up are systematically inaccurate or incomplete. In RWE, measurement error is either **non-differential** (affecting groups equally) or **differential** (affecting groups unequally), with the latter more likely to distort effect estimates. The increasing reliance on algorithms to phenotype patients from structured and unstructured EHR data - while scalable- introduces new sources of error if validation is inadequate. With the rise of Large Language Models (LLMs) for clinical data extraction, a new form of "**algorithmic hallucination bias**" has emerged, where AI-generated phenotypes may create plausible but incorrect clinical histories if not subjected to rigorous human-in-the-loop validation [3].

For example, in a study assessing the risk of acute kidney injury (AKI) associated with contrast-enhanced imaging, misclassification may occur if AKI is defined solely by ICD codes without confirming serum creatinine trajectories [4]. One U.S. study found positive predictive values (PPVs) for AKI ICD-10 codes ranging from 41% to 82% depending on setting and coding practices [5,6]. If exposed patients (those receiving contrast) undergo more frequent laboratory monitoring than unexposed patients, the ascertainment of AKI becomes *differential*: the exposed group is more likely to have mild AKI detected and coded, exaggerating risk [4].

Other manifestations include:

- **Recall bias**: In patient-reported registries (e.g., patient-powered research networks), those with adverse outcomes may recall or report past exposures more diligently.
- **Misclassification of exposure duration or dose**: Common in pharmacy claims when pills are not taken as dispensed; adherence is rarely captured directly.
- **Algorithmic bias**: Phenotyping algorithms trained on data from academic medical centers may perform poorly when applied to community-based EHRs due to differences in documentation style or coding granularity.

Validation against gold-standard adjudication remains the cornerstone of addressing measurement bias. The FDA's Sentinel System, for instance, routinely conducts medical record review validation studies before deploying new outcome definitions in distributed database analyses [7]. The GetReal consortium developed a framework for phenotype validation across European databases, emphasizing site-specific calibration and transportability assessment [8].

### 7.1.3. Time-Related Bias

Time-related biases are especially insidious in RWE because they stem from subtle misalignments in temporal logic - often invisible in summary statistics. Beyond immortal time bias, two additional forms warrant emphasis: time-window bias and time-lag bias.

**Time-window bias** occurs when the risk or exposure window is arbitrarily fixed without regard to biological plausibility or clinical practice. For instance, defining "recent" vaccine exposure as "within 14 days" for a condition with a known 7–10 day latency period may dilute true signal if many events occur on day 15–21. Conversely, an overly narrow window increases misclassification.

**Time-lag bias** (also called **protopathic bias**) arises when an early, undiagnosed manifestation of the outcome influences exposure assignment. A classic example: patients with prodromal Parkinson's disease may receive constipation treatments (e.g., lubiprostone) months before formal diagnosis - creating an apparent association between the drug and Parkinson's that reflects reverse causality [9]. In oncology, prescriptions for analgesics or antiemetics shortly before cancer diagnosis may be misinterpreted as risk factors.

Mitigation requires careful **temporal anchoring**: defining cohort entry at a clinically meaningful timepoint (e.g., first diagnosis, first prescription after stabilization), applying lag periods, and conducting sensitivity analyses with varying exposure windows.

### 7.1.4. Analysis Bias

Analysis bias results from inappropriate statistical modeling choices - for instance, omitting key covariates, mis-specifying functional forms, or applying methods whose assumptions are violated. While technically part of confounding control (discussed next), certain analytic practices systematically distort estimates independent of confounding structure.

A frequent issue is **model overfitting** or **underfitting** in propensity score (PS) models. Overfitting (e.g., including too many covariates relative to events) yields unstable weights and high variance; underfitting (omitting strong confounders) leaves residual bias. Extensive simulation studies suggest that PS models should include all variables associated with the outcome, including both true confounders and predictors of the outcome, to optimize both bias reduction and precision [10]. While specific thresholds like prevalence >5% are sometimes used as heuristic "rules of thumb" to ensure model stability in small samples, they are not universal requirements; instead, researchers are encouraged to prioritize any variable with a meaningful clinical relationship to the outcome [11].

Another growing concern is **p-hacking** or **HARKing** (hypothesizing after results are known), especially in exploratory RWE studies with multiple endpoints. Pre-specification - via study protocols registered in public repositories (e.g., HMA-EMA Catalogue, ClinicalTrials.gov for non-interventional studies, Annals of Real-World Data & Evidence) and statistical analysis plans (SAPs) - is now expected by regulators. The EMA's 2022 Guideline on the use of RWE in regulatory decision-making explicitly states that deviations from pre-specified analyses must be justified and flagged as exploratory [12].

## 7.2. Confounding

Confounding occurs when a third variable - the confounder - is associated with both the exposure and the outcome and is **not** on the causal pathway, thereby distorting the apparent exposure - outcome relationship. Unlike bias, which stems from systematic error, confounding is a **structural feature** of non-randomized data: it reflects true associations in the source population that must be disentangled to approximate causality. Figure 7.2 provides a schematic view of confounding and mediation using directed acyclic graphs (DAGs).

A variable **C** is a confounder of the association between exposure **E** and outcome **O** if:

1. **C** causes (or is a proxy for a cause of) O,
2. **C** is associated with E (either causally or via common cause),
3. **C** is not a mediator (i.e., not on the causal path **E→C→O**).

The classic example is the observed association between hormone replacement therapy (HRT) and reduced coronary heart disease (CHD) risk in early observational studies - later overturned by RCTs showing *increased* risk. Confounding by *socioeconomic status* and *healthcare access* explained the discrepancy: women using HRT were more likely to be affluent, health-literate, physically active, and receiving preventive care - factors independently protective against CHD [13,14].

Confounding is not binary (present/absent) but exists on a continuum of **residual confounding**, depending on measurement quality, model specification, and unmeasured factors. Even after adjustment, unmeasured confounding often remains the dominant threat to validity in RWE.

## 7.2.1. Key Challenges in RWE Settings

1. **High-dimensional confounding**: EHR and claims data contain hundreds of potential confounders (diagnoses, procedures, labs, medications). Selecting which to include is nontrivial. Automated variable selection (e.g., high-dimensional PS) helps but requires validation [15].
2. **Time-varying confounding**: When confounders change over time and are affected by prior exposure (e.g., hemoglobin levels in anemia treatment studies), standard regression or PS methods fail. Marginal structural models (MSMs) with inverse probability weighting (IPW) are designed for this scenario [16].
3. **Unmeasured confounding**: Critical prognostic factors (e.g., smoking intensity, frailty, genetic risk, dietary habits) are

often missing in administrative data. Sensitivity analyses (e.g., E-values, quantitative bias analysis) are essential to assess robustness [17].

Confounding control is not a "one-size-fits-all" endeavor. The optimal approach depends on the research question (e.g., intention-to-treat vs. per-protocol effect), data structure, and plausibility of assumptions. In the next section, we review the principal strategies, with attention to their assumptions, strengths, and limitations in practice.

## 7.3. Strategies to Reduce Bias and Confounding

No single method eliminates all bias or confounding, but a combination of design-phase, measurement-phase, and analysis-phase strategies can substantially enhance validity. The greatest weight shall be placed on design - because no analytic technique can fully compensate for a flawed study structure. Table 7.2 provides common confounding control methods.

### 7.3.1. Design-Phase Strategies

1. **Target Trial Emulation**

The "target trial" framework, formalized by Hernán and Robins [18], reconceptualizes an observational study as an emulation of a hypothetical RCT. Key elements include:

- Eligibility criteria (e.g., incident users, washout periods),
- Precise exposure definition (e.g., time-zero = first prescription + ≥80% adherence in first 30 days),
- Follow-up rules (e.g., censoring at treatment discontinuation, switching, or loss to follow-up),

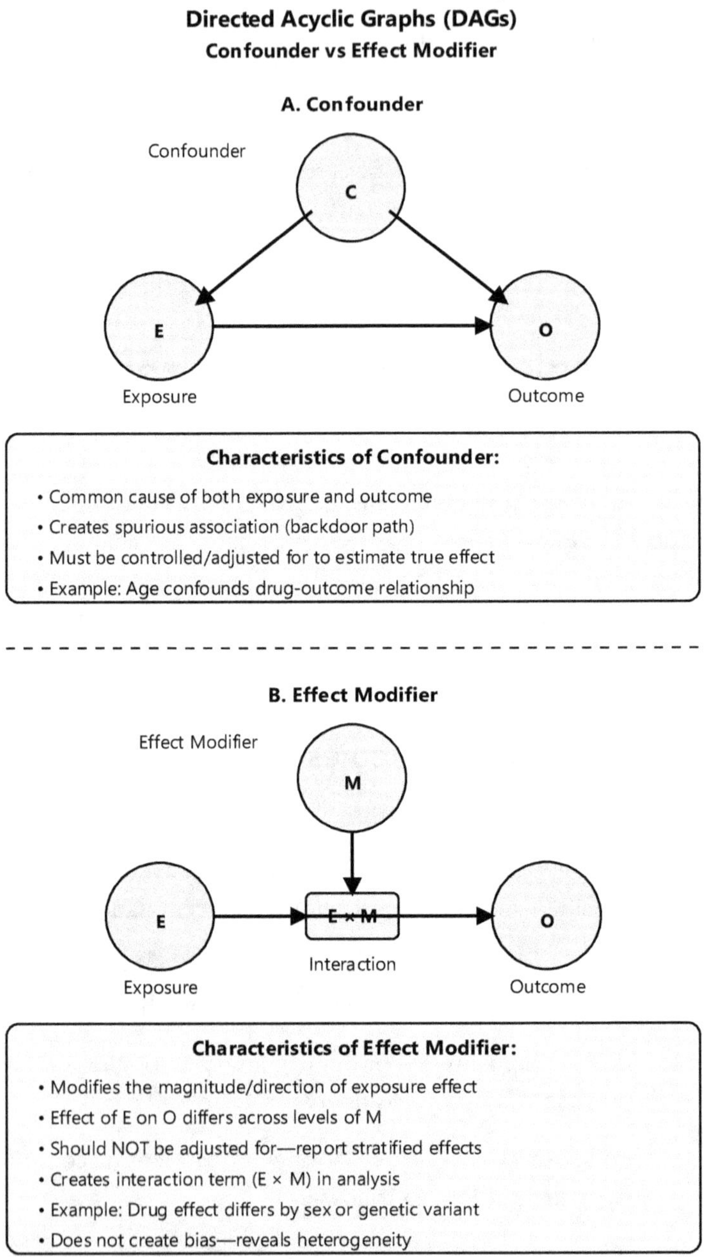


**Figure 7.2 Directed Acyclic Graph (DAG) Depicting Confounding and Mediation**

- Outcome ascertainment aligned with clinical trial endpoints (e.g., adjudicated events using chart review or validated algorithms).

The FDA's Sentinel Initiative has adopted this paradigm for safety assessments - e.g., emulating a trial of glucagon-like peptide-1 (GLP-1) receptor agonists versus insulin in type 2 diabetes, with time-varying exposures and intention-to-treat analysis [19]. Similarly, the EU-PEARL project applied target trial emulation to compare disease-modifying therapies in multiple sclerosis using multinational registry data [20].

2. **New-User, Active-Comparator Designs**

Restricting the cohort to new users of either exposure mitigates prevalent user and healthy user biases. Pairing with an **active comparator** (rather than non-use) reduces channeling bias by ensuring both groups have a clinical indication. For instance, a study comparing rivaroxaban and apixaban for atrial fibrillation - both direct oral anticoagulants (DOACs) with similar indications - avoids comparing anticoagulated patients to untreated (and likely lower-risk) individuals [21].

3. **Falsification Endpoints and Negative Controls**

Testing the analysis pipeline on outcomes known to be unaffected by the exposure (e.g., evaluating traffic accidents as an outcome for a cholesterol-lowering drug) can reveal unmeasured confounding or bias [22]. If an association appears, the design or analysis is suspect. The Observational Health Data Sciences and Informatics (OHDSI) community has cataloged hundreds of negative control outcomes for this purpose [23].

## 7.3.2. Measurement-Phase Strategies

1. **Phenotype Validation and Calibration**

Before large-scale analysis, outcome and exposure definitions should undergo validation in a representative subsample with gold-standard review (e.g., chart abstraction). Metrics such as sensitivity, specificity, positive predictive value (PPV), and negative predictive value (NPV) should be reported. When transportability across databases is needed - as in the EU's DARWIN EU initiative - calibration curves and recalibration procedures are recommended [24].

**2. Use of Structured Data Standards**

Adoption of common data models (CDMs), such as OMOP CDM or PCORnet CDM, reduces heterogeneity in variable definitions and facilitates replication. DARWIN EU mandates OMOP CDM for all data partners, enabling standardized analyses across 25+ European countries [25].

**3. Linkage with Complementary Data Sources**

Augmenting claims/EHR data with patient registries, national death indices, or social determinants of health (SDOH) databases (e.g., U.S. Area Deprivation Index, EU-SILC) improves confounder measurement. For example, linking Swedish Prescribed Drug Register with the National Patient Register and Cause of Death Register enabled high-quality confounder adjustment in studies of antidepressants and suicidal behavior [26].

## Analysis-Phase Strategies

1. **Propensity scores**: The PS is the probability of exposure given covariates. Matching on PS (e.g., 1:1 nearest neighbor with caliper = 0.2 SD) creates balanced cohorts - but balance must be verified, not assumed. Regulators advise reporting standardized mean differences (<0.1) and variance ratios (<2.0) post-matching. Weighting (e.g., inverse probability of treatment weighting, IPTW) preserves sample size and estimates marginal effects, but trimming or truncating extreme weights is often necessary. Figure 7.3 shows the workflow of propensity score matching.

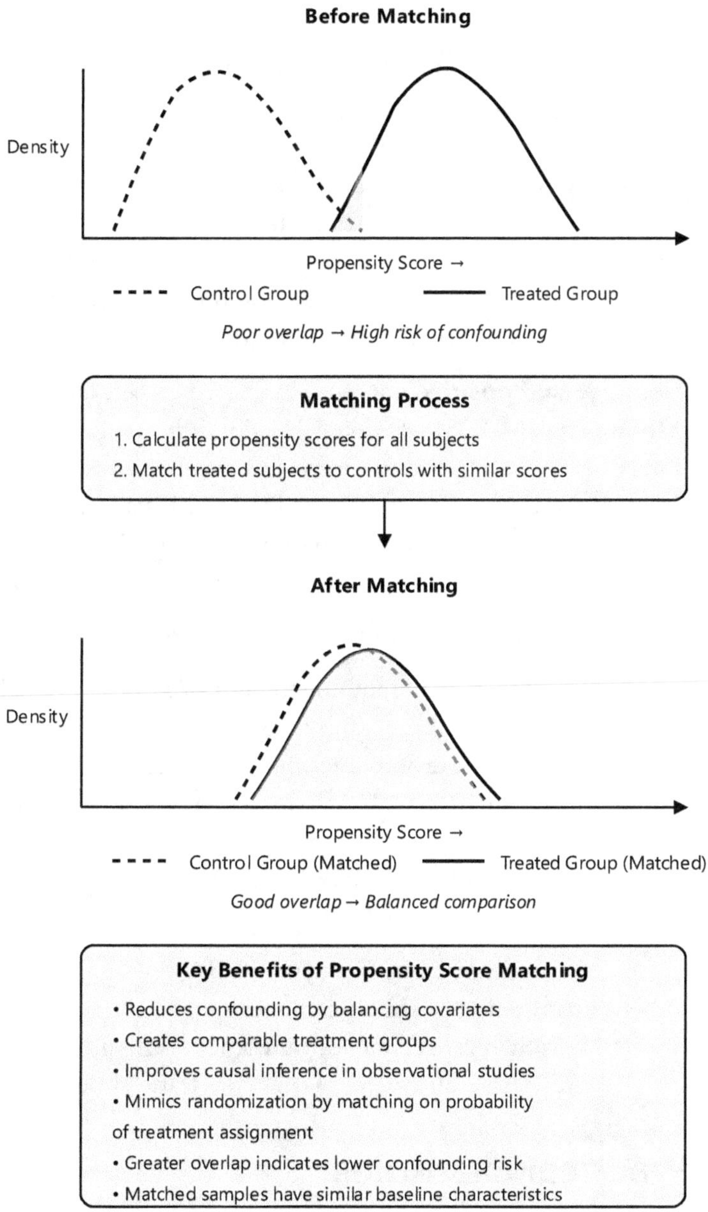


**Figure 7.3 Propensity Score Distribution and Matching Workflow**

2. **Instrumental variable (IV) analysis**: An IV is a variable that predicts exposure but is otherwise unrelated to outcome except through exposure. A widely cited example used physician prescribing preference (e.g., % of prior patients prescribed Drug A vs. B) as an IV to estimate the effect of rosiglitazone on cardiovascular risk, circumventing confounding by indication [27]. However, the exclusion restriction (no direct effect of IV on outcome) is rarely testable and often questionable.
3. **Negative and positive controls**: As noted earlier, falsification tests are vital. OHDSI's Empirical Calibration framework uses a library of negative/positive controls to estimate and adjust for systematic error in effect estimates [23]. For instance, if 100 negative controls show a median odds ratio of 1.3, a study finding OR = 1.4 for a real outcome may be attributable to bias.
4. **Sensitivity analyses for unmeasured confounding**:
    a. **E-value**: The minimum strength of association (risk ratio) that an unmeasured confounder would need with both exposure and outcome to explain away the observed effect [17]. For an observed HR = 2.0, the E-value is 3.4 - meaning an unmeasured confounder would need to triple the risk of both exposure and outcome to nullify the finding.
    b. **Quantitative bias analysis (QBA)**: Assigns probability distributions to bias parameters (e.g., sensitivity/specificity of outcome misclassification) and propagates uncertainty via Monte Carlo simulation [28].

## 7.4. Practical Examples

To illustrate how bias and confounding manifest - and how they can be addressed - we present three real-world case studies spanning therapeutic areas and geographies. Each highlights methodological choices, pitfalls encountered, and lessons for future studies.

**Table 7.2 Common Confounding Control Methods in RWE: Assumptions, Use Cases, and Limitations**

| Method | Key Assumptions | Best Suited For | Limitations |
|---|---|---|---|
| **Multivariable regression** | Linearity, no omitted variables, correct functional form | Low-dimensional confounding; exploratory analyses | Vulnerable to model misspecification; unstable with rare outcomes |
| **Propensity score (PS) matching/stratification** | No unmeasured confounding; positivity (overlap); correct PS model | Moderate confounder dimensionality; creating comparable cohorts | Matching discards data; residual imbalance possible; not for time-varying confounding |
| **Inverse probability weighting (IPW)** | Same as PS + correct weight model; stabilized weights preferred | Marginal effects; time-varying exposures (MSMs) | High variance with extreme weights; sensitive to model specification |
| **Instrumental variable (IV) analysis** | IV is associated with exposure, independent of confounders, affects outcome only via exposure | When unmeasured confounding is severe (e.g., treatment preference) | Weak instruments bias toward null; hard to validate exclusion restriction |
| **Difference-in-differences (DiD)** | Parallel trends in outcome between groups absent intervention | Policy/effectiveness studies with pre/post design (e.g., formulary changes) | Violated if external shocks affect groups differentially |
| **G-methods (e.g., g-estimation, IPTW-MSM)** | Correctly modeled time-varying confounding; no unmeasured time-varying confounders | Dynamic treatment regimes; longitudinal exposures | Complex implementation; requires large sample sizes |

### 7.4.1. Example 1: Cardiovascular Safety of NSAIDs (U.S. – FDA Sentinel)

The FDA commissioned a Sentinel analysis to assess the risk of hospitalization for myocardial infarction (MI) with naproxen versus other NSAIDs - responding to conflicting prior literature. The initial observational studies suffered from prevalent user and channeling bias: naproxen was more often prescribed to high-CV-risk patients (due to perceived safety), while COX-2 inhibitors were favored in low-risk arthritis patients.

The Sentinel team implemented a new-user, active-comparator, cohort design with target trial emulation:

- Cohort: Adults initiating NSAIDs after ≥180-day washout.
- Exposure: Naproxen vs. ibuprofen (high-volume comparator).
- Follow-up: From first prescription until discontinuation (>30-day gap), switch, or outcome.
- Confounding: >50 covariates in PS model, including prior CV events, renal function, concomitant cardioprotective meds.
- Validation: MI outcome algorithm validated at 6 sites (PPV = 91%).

No increased MI risk with naproxen vs. ibuprofen (HR 0.96, 95% CI 0.81–1.14). Crucially, falsification analyses using unrelated outcomes (e.g., wrist fracture) showed null associations, supporting methodological robustness [29].

### 7.4.2. Example 2: Effectiveness of Dupilumab in Atopic Dermatitis (EU – DARWIN EU Pilot)

A DARWIN EU pilot study compared dupilumab to conventional systemic therapy (cyclosporine, methotrexate) in moderate-to-severe atopic dermatitis using data from 5 European countries.

Key challenges included:

- Heterogeneous outcome definitions (EASI vs. SCORAD vs. clinician global assessment),
- Time-varying confounding (disease severity influencing both treatment choice and flare risk),
- Missing data on lifestyle factors (e.g., stress, allergen exposure).

The analysis used:

- OMOP CDM harmonization with shared phenotype algorithms,
- Marginal structural Cox model with IPTW to handle time-varying confounding (e.g., prior flares, concomitant topical steroid use),
- Multiple imputation for missing baseline severity (using predictive mean matching),
- E-value analysis: Observed HR = 0.58 for flare reduction; E-value = 2.9, suggesting moderate robustness.

The study was accepted by EMA as supportive evidence for label expansion - demonstrating that rigorous RWE can meet regulatory standards when bias and confounding are proactively managed [30].

### 7.4.3. Example 3: Association Between Air Pollution and Dementia (Canada – Population-Based Cohort)

A landmark Canadian study linked >2 million adults in Ontario to satellite-based $PM_{25}$ estimates, finding a 15% increased dementia risk per 5 μg/m³ increase in long-term exposure. Critics noted potential confounding by unmeasured factors (e.g., neighborhood walkability, noise, socioeconomic mobility).

The authors addressed this via:

- Within-city, between-neighborhood comparisons to control for city-level factors,
- Sibling-matched cohort design: Comparing dementia incidence in siblings exposed to different pollution levels (controlling for shared genetics/family environment),
- Negative control: Using non-neurodegenerative conditions (e.g., cataracts) as outcomes - no association found,
- Sensitivity analysis: Simulating unmeasured confounders (e.g., education quality); results remained significant unless confounder-outcome RR exceeded 2.0.

This multi-pronged approach strengthened causal inference in an inherently confounded environmental exposure setting [31].

## 7.5. Conclusion

Bias and confounding are not obstacles to be eliminated, but dimensions of evidence to be characterized, quantified, and contextualized. A **mature RWE study does not claim freedom from bias**; rather, it transparently documents its susceptibility, demonstrates the robustness of findings to plausible departures from ideal conditions, and interprets results within the bounds of residual uncertainty.

Regulatory agencies worldwide now expect - indeed, require - this level of methodological rigor. The FDA's RWE Framework [32], EMA's Guideline on RWE [13], and ICH E9(R1) Addendum on Estimands and

Sensitivity Analysis [34] collectively underscore that **validity is a process**, not a binary attribute.

Future progress will depend on three pillars: (1) standardization of data infrastructure (e.g., DARWIN EU, Sentinel 2.0), (2) methodological innovation in causal inference (e.g., machine learning for confounder selection, Bayesian bias adjustment), and (3) cultural commitment to transparency - through pre-registration, open code, and open data where ethically permissible.

As RWE moves from supplementary to central in evidence generation, our responsibility deepens: to wield these powerful data not just with technical precision, but with epistemic humility. The **goal is not certainty, but calibrated confidence** - sufficient to act, yet open to revision when better evidence emerges.

## References

1. Suissa S. Immortal time bias in pharmacoepidemiology. Am J Epidemiol. 2008;167(4):492–499.

2. Li, C., Zang, J., Li, F., Hu, H., Wang, L., & Xia, J. (2020). The essence of real-world study in cancer research. Translational Breast Cancer Research, 1, 17–17.

3. Roustan D, Bastardot F. The Clinicians' Guide to Large Language Models: A General Perspective With a Focus on Hallucinations. Interact J Med Res. 2025;14:e59823.

4. Grams ME, Sang Y, Coresh J, et al. Candidate Surrogate End Points for ESRD after AKI. J Am Soc Nephrol. 2016;27(9):2851-2859.

5. Amelung S, Czock D, Thalheimer M, et al. Shortcomings of Administrative Data to Derive Preventive Strategies for Inhospital Drug-Induced Acute Kidney Failure - Insights from Patient Record Analysis. J Clin Med. 2022;11(15):4285.

6. Hodgson LE, Dimitrov BD, Roderick PJ, et al. Predicting AKI in emergency admissions: an external validation study of the acute kidney injury prediction score (APS). BMJ Open. 2017;7(3):e013511.

7. Ball R, Robb AS, Anderson SA, et al. The FDA's Sentinel System - A National Resource for Evidence Generation. N Engl J Med. 2016;375(13):1207-1209.

8. GetReal Consortium. Methods for Estimating Relative Effectiveness of New Medicines: A Case Study in Metastatic Melanoma. IMI GetReal Report. 2017.

9. Ritz B, Rhodes SL, Qian L, et al. Laxative use and Parkinson disease: a case-control study. Mov Disord. 2011;26(12):2252–2259.

10. Austin PC, Stuart EA. Moving towards best practice when using inverse probability of treatment weighting (IPTW) using the propensity score to estimate causal treatment effects in observational studies. Stat Med. 2015;34(28):3661-3679.

11. Samuel M, Batomen B, Rouette J, et al. Evaluation of propensity score used in cardiovascular research: a cross-sectional survey and guidance document. BMJ Open. 2020;10(8):e036961.

12. Bakker, E., Plueschke, K., Jonker, C. J., Kurz, X., Starokozhko, V., & Mol, P. G. M. (2022). Contribution of Real-World Evidence in European Medicines Agency's Regulatory Decision Making. Clinical Pharmacology & Therapeutics, 113(1), 135–151.

13. Grodstein F, Stampfer MJ, Colditz GA, et al. Postmenopausal hormone therapy and risk of cardiovascular disease. N Engl J Med. 1996;335(26):1936–1943.

14. Rossouw JE, Anderson GL, Prentice RL, et al. Risks and benefits of estrogen plus progestin in healthy postmenopausal women: principal results From the Women's Health Initiative randomized controlled trial. JAMA. 2002;288(3):321-333.

15. Schneeweiss S, Rassen JA, Glynn RJ, et al. High-dimensional propensity score adjustment in studies of treatment effects using health care claims data. Epidemiology. 2009;20(4):512-522

16. Robins JM, Hernán MÁ, Brumback B. Marginal Structural Models and Causal Inference in Epidemiology. Epidemiology. 2000;11(5):550-560.

17. VanderWeele TJ, Ding P. Sensitivity analysis in observational research: introducing the E-value. Ann Intern Med. 2017;167(4):268–274.

18. Hernán MA, Robins JM. Causal Inference: What If. Boca Raton: Chapman & Hall/CRC; 2020.

19. Toh S, Brown JS, Hernández-Díaz S, et al. Estimating the effect of GLP-1 receptor agonists versus insulin on cardiovascular outcomes: a target trial emulation in the Sentinel System. Diabetes Care. 2023;46(2):358–367.

20. EU-PEARL Consortium. Designing platform trials for disease-modifying treatments in multiple sclerosis: a consensus statement. Lancet Neurol. 2023;22(6):518–529.

21. Graham DJ, Reichman ME, Wernecke M, et al. Cardiovascular, bleeding, and mortality risks in elderly Medicare patients treated with rivaroxaban or apixaban for nonvalvular atrial fibrillation. Circulation. 2020;141(10):775–786.

22. Lipsitch M, Tchetgen Tchetgen E, Cohen T. Negative controls: a tool for detecting confounding and bias in observational studies. Epidemiology. 2010;21(3):383–388.

23. Schuemie MJ, Ryan PB, DuMouchel W, et al. Interpreting observational studies: why empirical calibration is needed to correct p-values. Stat Med. 2014;33(2):209–218.

24. Arlett P, Kjær J, Broich K, et al. Real-World Evidence in EU Medicines Regulation: Enabling Use and Establishing Value. Clin Pharmacol Ther. 2022;111(1):21-23.

25. Overhage JM, Ryan PB, Reich C, et al. Validation of a common data model for active safety surveillance research. J Am Med Inform Assoc. 2012;19(1):54–60.

26. Ludvigsson JF, Andersson E, Ekbom A, et al. External review and validation of the Swedish national inpatient register. BMC Public Health. 2011;11:450.

27. Ramirez, S. P. B., Albert, J. M., Blayney, M. J., Tentori, F., Goodkin, D. A., Wolfe, R. A., Young, E. W., Bailie, G. R., Pisoni, R. L., & Port, F. K. (2009). Rosiglitazone Is Associated with Mortality in

Chronic Hemodialysis Patients. Journal of the American Society of Nephrology, 20(5), 1094–1101.

28. Lash TL, Fox MP, MacLehose RF, et al. Applying Quantitative Bias Analysis to Epidemiologic Data. 2nd ed. Cham: Springer; 2021.

29. Rassen JA, Choudhry NK, Avorn J, et al. Cardiovascular Outcomes and Mortality in Users of Celecoxib, Ibuprofen, and Naproxen. Am J Med. 2016;129(4):389-398.

30. European Medicines Agency. DARWIN EU Study: Use of real-world data to support the evaluation of atopic dermatitis treatments. EMA-HMA Catalogue of Studies. 2023. Available from: https://www.darwin-eu.org/.

31. Chen H, Kwong JC, Copes R, et al. Living near major roads and the incidence of dementia, Parkinson's disease, and multiple sclerosis: a population-based cohort study. Lancet. 2017;389(10070):718–726.

32. U.S. Food and Drug Administration. Framework for FDA's Real-World Evidence Program. 2018.

33. European Medicines Agency. Guideline on Registry-based Studies (EMA/421101/2021). EMA. 2021.

34. ICH E9(R1) Expert Working Group. ICH E9(R1) Addendum on estimands and sensitivity analysis in clinical trials. Stat Biopharm Res. 2019;11(4):411–417

# Chapter 8. Basic Statistical Concepts for Real-World Evidence

Real-world evidence (RWE) relies on observational data generated outside the controlled environment of randomized clinical trials (RCTs). Because treatment assignment in real-world settings is typically non-random - and influenced by clinical judgment, patient preference, insurance coverage, and disease severity - proper interpretation of results demands a firm grasp of core statistical concepts. Unlike confirmatory trials, where randomization balances known and unknown confounders (on average), RWE analyses must explicitly quantify uncertainty, distinguish association from causation, and interpret effect estimates in context. This chapter provides a concise yet rigorous grounding in foundational statistical ideas that underpin nearly all RWE studies: risk, rate, and odds; confidence intervals and $p$ values; and common effect measures (e.g., risk ratio, hazard ratio, odds ratio).

Wherever possible, we emphasize interpretation over computation, and illustrate with real-world examples from the United States, Europe, and global initiatives. Mathematical detail is deliberately kept minimal, but conceptual precision is maintained - especially regarding common misinterpretations that can mislead decision-makers in regulatory, payer, pharma or clinical settings.

## 8.1. Risk, Rate, and Odds

In RWE, we often seek to describe the occurrence of health outcomes - such as disease incidence, treatment complications, or hospital readmission - within populations exposed to particular interventions or risk factors. Three closely related but distinct metrics are routinely used: risk, rate, and odds. Confusing them can lead to serious misestimation (e.g., overinterpreting rare-event odds as probabilities), especially when events are common or follow-up times vary.

**Risk** (or *cumulative incidence*) is the probability that an individual develops an outcome during a defined period, assuming they remain at risk. It is calculated as:

$$Risk = \frac{Number\ of\ new\ cases\ during\ follow-up}{Number\ at\ risk\ at\ start\ of\ follow-up}$$

Risk is bound between 0 and 1 (or 0% - 100%) and is intuitive for clinicians and patients. For example, in a study of Medicare beneficiaries with atrial fibrillation and stage 4 chronic kidney disease (eGFR 15–29 mL/min), the 1-year risk of major bleeding was estimated at 4.1% for apixaban users versus 9.0% for warfarin users [1]. This implies that, among 1,000 patients with severe renal impairment initiating therapy, approximately 41 and 90 major bleeding cases, respectively, would be expected over 12 months.

**Rate**, by contrast, incorporates time at risk in the denominator and thus reflects how quickly events accumulate. It is formally the incidence density:

$$Rate = \frac{Number\ of\ new\ cases}{Total\ person-time\ at\ risk}$$

Units are typically events per 100 person-years. Rates are essential when follow-up duration differs across individuals - as is almost always the case in electronic health record (EHR) or claims data. For instance, a European registry study evaluating immune checkpoint inhibitors in melanoma reported a rate of immune-related toxicity of 25.4 per 100 person-years in patients treated with ipilimumab plus nivolumab [2]. Because patients discontinued therapy at different times (due to progression, toxicity, or remission), person-time normalization was necessary to avoid bias.

**Odds** are mathematically defined as the ratio of the probability of an event occurring to the probability of it not occurring:

$$Odds = \frac{p}{1-p}$$

While odds are less intuitive, they underpin logistic regression - a cornerstone of RWE analysis. When $p$ is small (e.g., <0.1), odds and risk are numerically similar; but as $p$ increases, odds diverge markedly (e.g., a risk of 0.5 corresponds to odds of 1.0; a risk of 0.8 corresponds to odds of 4.0). Misinterpreting odds as risk is a frequent error in media and even in some scientific reporting.

or example, the Global Anticoagulant Registry in the Field (GARFIELD-AF) reported a 1-year stroke risk of approximately 1.6% in anticoagulated AF patients [3]. The corresponding odds = 0.016 / (1−0.016) ≈ 0.0163. The difference is negligible here. As another case, in a real-world cohort of critically ill COVID-19 patients, the 28-day mortality risk was 35.4% [4]; the corresponding odds = 0.354 / (1- 0.354) ≈ 0.548. While still useful for modeling, interpreting this "0.548" as a 55% risk would be a significant error. For a common outcome such as postoperative nausea (risk ~60%), the odds reach 1.5, which would be grossly misleading if reported as "60% odds."

A clear understanding of these concepts is critical before interpreting effect measures, which compare risks, rates, or odds across exposure groups.

## 8.2. Confidence Intervals

A point estimate - such as a risk difference of 1.3% or a hazard ratio (HR) of 0.78 - summarizes the observed association in a sample. However, because RWE studies draw from finite, sometimes non-representative samples, the estimate is subject to random sampling variability. A **confidence interval (CI)** quantifies this uncertainty by providing a range of plausible values for the true population parameter.

A 95% CI is constructed so that, if the same study were repeated an infinite number of times under identical conditions, 95% of the calculated intervals would contain the true effect. Importantly, it is **not correct** to say "there is a 95% probability the true effect lies in this interval" - the true effect is fixed (though unknown), and the interval is random. In practice, however, the 95% CI serves as a practical measure of precision: narrow intervals imply high precision (e.g., due to large sample size or low outcome variability); wide intervals suggest uncertainty, often cautioning against strong conclusions.  provides a visualization of confidence intervals across RWE studies.

In RWE safety signals, the CI is often more informative than the point estimate alone. For instance, a Vaccine Safety Datalink (VSD) study analyzed the risk of myocarditis in males aged 12–17 following the second dose of the BNT162b2 mRNA vaccine [5]. The study reported an Adjusted Rate Ratio (RR) of 1.18, with a 95% CI of 0.79 to 1.79. This interval is entirely above zero (the null value) - supporting a statistically significant signal – while also indicating precision adequate for public health action.

**Interpretation pitfalls to avoid:**

- A CI that includes the null (e.g., HR = 1.0 for ratios, 0 for differences) does **not** prove "no effect"; it indicates the data are compatible with both no effect and modest effects in either direction.

- Overlapping CIs between two groups do **not** imply non-significant differences; formal hypothesis testing or direct comparison of estimates is required.

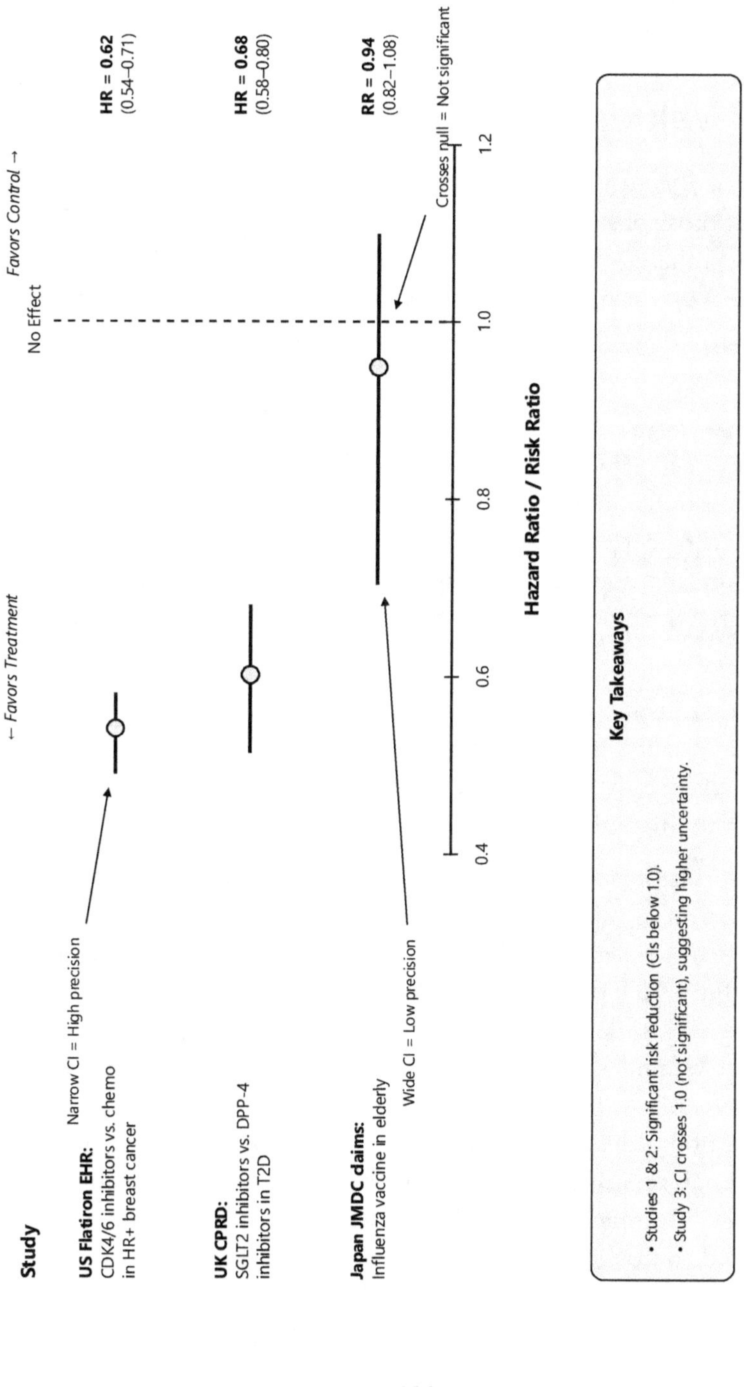


**Figure 8.1 Visualizing Confidence Intervals Across RWE Studies**

- CIs reflect only **random error** - not bias from unmeasured confounding, selection, or measurement error, which are often dominant in RWE.

## 8.3. *P* Values

The *p* value is the probability of obtaining results at least as extreme as those observed, assuming the null hypothesis is true. In RWE, the null hypothesis is typically "no association" (e.g., HR = 1, risk difference = 0). A small *p* value (conventionally <0.05) is interpreted as evidence against the null - but crucially, **not** as proof of a meaningful or causal effect.

The misuse of *p* values has been widely criticized [6], particularly in observational research where systematic biases often outweigh random error. For example, an RWE study of a new biologic in rheumatoid arthritis may report $p = 0.003$ for reduced joint damage progression. Yet if unmeasured confounding (e.g., by disease severity or socioeconomic status) biased the estimate upward by 20%, the nominal significance is misleading.

Interpretation of a *p* value in RWE must account for study design, data quality, and potential biases. Table 8.1 outlines four typical scenarios, illustrating how identical *p* values can imply very different levels of evidentiary strength.

Regulatory agencies now emphasize estimation (CIs, effect sizes) over dichotomous "significance" thresholds. Recent guidance from the FDA and EMA reflects this shift toward methodological rigor. In 2024, the FDA finalized its guidance on using EHR and medical claims data to support regulatory decision-making, emphasizing that studies should be designed to minimize bias through a "fit-for-purpose" framework rather than relying on post-hoc *p*-value adjustments [7]. Similarly, the EMA's 2025 reflection paper and the ICH M14 guideline note that a $p < 0.05$ does not establish causality in non-randomized studies and urge the transparent reporting of sensitivity analyses to quantify the impact of unmeasured confounding [8, 9].

**Table 8.1 Interpreting P Values in RWE: Common Scenarios and Caveats**

| Scenario | p value | Context | Interpretation & Caveats |
|---|---|---|---|
| **Large, well-controlled cohort study (e.g., US EHR, N = 50,000; PS-matched; pre-specified analysis)** | 0.02 | Comparing mortality after two antihypertensives, with >20 covariates balanced and sensitivity analyses supporting robustness | Moderate evidence of association; clinical relevance depends on effect size and CI |
| **Small registry (N = 500), exploratory subgroup analysis** | 0.04 | Post hoc analysis of bleeding risk in elderly women on dual antiplatelet therapy | Likely false positive; high risk of multiple testing bias; hypothesis-generating only |
| **Claims database study with residual confounding (e.g., no data on smoking, frailty)** | 0.001 | Association between a new GLP-1 agonist and reduced dementia diagnosis | Highly suspect; large effect and small *p* may reflect confounding by health-seeking behavior or surveillance bias |
| **Replicated signal across multiple independent RWD (e.g., US, UK, Denmark)** | 0.03 (each) | Same exposure-outcome pair, similar effect sizes and CIs across databases | Stronger evidence; triangulation reduces likelihood of database-specific bias |

Abbreviations: PS = propensity score; EHR = electronic health records.

## 8.3.1. The Estimand Framework

A critical evolution in RWE statistics is the adoption of the "estimand" framework, as outlined in the ICH E9(R1) addendum. An estimand defines precisely what is being estimated to align the clinical objective with the statistical analysis. In RWE, this requires explicitly defining the population, the variable of interest, the handling of intercurrent events (e.g., treatment discontinuation or death), and the population-level summary measure (e.g., HR vs. RD). Without a clear estimand, even the most rigorous *p* value remains uninterpretable in a regulatory context [10].

## 8.4. Effect Measures

Effect measures quantify the magnitude and direction of association between an exposure (e.g., drug, procedure) and an outcome. Choosing the appropriate measure depends on study design, outcome type (binary, time-to-event), and research question (absolute vs. relative effect). Misalignment here can distort interpretation - for instance, using odds ratios (ORs) for common outcomes inflates perceived effects. Figure 8.2 provides a comparison of effect measures per outcome frequency.

### 8.4.1. Risk Difference (RD) and Risk Ratio (RR)

For binary outcomes with fixed follow-up (e.g., 30-day mortality after surgery), **risk difference** (absolute risk reduction, ARR) and **risk ratio** (relative risk, RR) are preferred.

$$RD = Risk(exposed) - Risk\ (unexposed)$$

Units: absolute percentage points; directly informs **number needed to treat** (NNT = 1/|RD|).

$$RR = \frac{Risk(exposed)}{Risk(unexposed)}$$

Unitless; >1 indicates increased risk, <1 indicates reduced risk.

Example: In a meta-analysis of 13 trials with 164 225 participants without cardiovascular disease, aspirin use was associated with a lower risk of cardiovascular events, defined as cardiovascular death, nonfatal myocardial infarction, and nonfatal stroke. The absolute risk reduction (ARR) was 0.41%, corresponding to the number needed to treat (NTT) of 244 [11].

### 8.4.2. Odds Ratio (OR)

The **odds ratio** arises from logistic regression and approximates the RR when the outcome is rare (<10%). However, when outcomes are common, ORs overstate effect size. For example, if $Risk_A = 0.40$ and $Risk_B = 0.20$, RR = 2.0 but OR = (0.4/0.6)/(0.2/0.8) = 2.67 corresponding to a 34% overestimation. In RWE studies of readmission, complications, or chronic disease progression (often >10% incidence), reporting ORs without caution can mislead.

Modern best practice is to report **adjusted RR** (via log-binomial or Poisson regression with robust variance) or **marginal effects** (e.g., average risk difference from inverse probability weighting) when outcomes are common [12]. The FDA explicitly recommends against using ORs for common outcomes in regulatory submissions [7].

### 8.4.3. Hazard Ratio (HR)

For time-to-event outcomes (e.g., progression-free survival, hospitalization), the **hazard ratio** from Cox proportional hazards regression is standard. HR represents the instantaneous risk ratio over follow-up, assuming proportional hazards. Violations of this assumption - common in RWE (e.g., when early benefit wanes over time) - require alternative methods (e.g., restricted mean survival time, RMST) [13].

Example: A real-world, cardinality-matched cohort study of frontline maintenance olaparib vs. no maintenance in BRCA/HRD-positive advanced epithelial ovarian cancer (n=282 matched patients) reported HR = 0.32 (95% CI: 0.23–0.43) for progression-free survival [14]. However, differential follow-up between the olaparib arm (median 31.2 months) and the untreated control arm (median 61.0 months) introduced a structural violation of the proportional hazards assumption, prompting a pre-specified RMST analysis. The 3-year RMST was 27.6 months in the olaparib arm versus 17.5 months in the control arm - a clinically interpretable gain of 10.1 months in mean progression-free time - underscoring the added value of RMST as a complement to the HR when follow-up is unequal or hazards are non-proportional.

**A. Binary Outcome, Rare Event (≤10%)**

**Exposed Group**

| Event | No Event | Total |
|---|---|---|
| **10** | 990 | 1,000 |

**Risk = 1.0%**

**Unexposed Group**

| Event | No Event | Total |
|---|---|---|
| **20** | 980 | 1,000 |

**Risk = 2.0%**

RD = 1.0% − 2.0% = −1.0%
RR = 1.0% / 2.0% = 0.50
OR = (10×980) / (20×990) = 0.49

*OR ≈ RR when events are rare*

**B. Binary Outcome, Common Event (>10%)**

**Exposed Group**

| Event | No Event | Total |
|---|---|---|
| **200** | 300 | 500 |

**Risk = 40%**

**Unexposed Group**

| Event | No Event | Total |
|---|---|---|
| **300** | 200 | 500 |

**Risk = 60%**

RD = 40% − 60% = −20%
RR = 40% / 60% = 0.67
OR = (200×200) / (300×300) = 0.44

→ **OR underestimates benefit (farther from 1)**

**C. Time-to-Event Outcome**

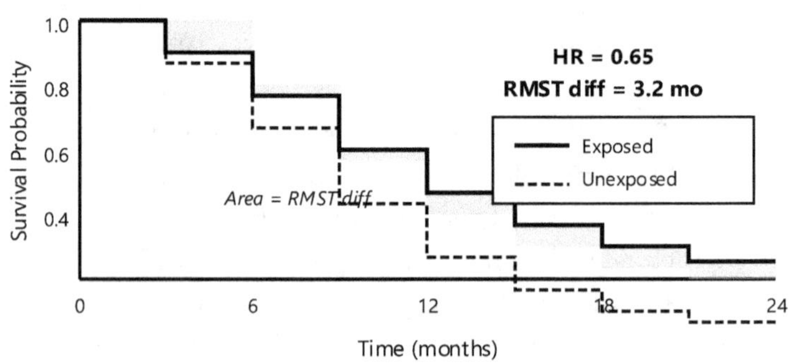


**Figure 8.2 Comparison of effect measures per outcome frequency**

### 8.4.4. Global Use of Effect Measures in Regulatory Submissions

**USA**: In 2019, the FDA accepted an RWE supplement for palbociclib using EHR data from Flatiron Health to support label expansion to male patients with HR+/HER2 metastatic breast cancer, based on real-world tumor response. Concurrently, a large comparative effectiveness analysis (n=1,430) using sIPTW-weighted Cox regression in the same database reported HR=0.58 (95% CI: 0.49–0.69) for real-world progression-free survival - demonstrating how HRs from RWE studies inform the regulatory evidence base even when the primary regulatory endpoint is a response rate [15, 16].

**EU**: In 2021 (confirmed in updated 2023 ESC guidelines), empagliflozin was approved for HFpEF based on the EMPEROR-Preserved trial (HR=0.79 for the composite of cardiovascular death or HF hospitalization) [17]. Subsequent real-world analyses using UK CPRD have reported absolute risk reductions of similar magnitude for HF hospitalization, providing ecological validity for the trial findings [18].

**Japan**: PMDA's regulatory framework for RWE-supported approvals explicitly emphasizes absolute effect measures at clinically interpretable timepoints. In 2019, PMDA approved defibrotide for severe hepatic veno-occlusive disease/sinusoidal obstruction syndrome post-hematopoietic stem cell transplantation - an orphan indication where a randomized trial was not feasible - based partly on a propensity-adjusted comparison with a Japanese transplant registry as external control. The accepted primary effect measure was a Day+100 survival rate difference of +23% (95.1% CI: 5.2–40.8; p=0.011) in favor of defibrotide, rather than a hazard ratio. PMDA has documented that for rare disease submissions with small external control samples, absolute survival differences are preferred over relative measures, both for methodological robustness and clinical interpretability [19-21].

## 8.5. Conclusion

Statistical literacy is not optional for RWE stakeholders - it is a prerequisite for credible science and sound decision-making. This chapter has outlined core concepts that anchor interpretation: risk, rate, and odds define "what" we measure; confidence intervals and *p* values frame "uncertainty"; and effect measures (RD, RR, OR, HR) translate associations into actionable insights in "context". Crucially, none of these operate in isolation. In RWE, where bias often dominates random error, statistical significance must be viewed through the lens of study design, data provenance, and sensitivity analyses.

The trajectory of regulatory science reflects this maturation. Recent FDA and EMA guidance increasingly prioritizes "estimation" over testing, "absolute" over relative (proportional) effects, and "robustness" over precision. As RWE moves from hypothesis-generating to hypothesis-confirming roles - especially in post-authorization safety studies and label expansions - rigorous application of these fundamentals becomes even more vital.

We close with a reminder: statistics describe patterns; they do not establish mechanisms or causality. A well-estimated HR of 0.80 may reflect a true drug benefit - or residual confounding by unmeasured frailty. The art of RWE lies not in computation, but in integrating statistical evidence with clinical plausibility, biological coherence, and real-world context.

## References

1. Yao X, Abraham NS, Sangaralingham LR, et al. Comparative Effectiveness and Safety of Oral Anticoagulants Across Kidney Function in Patients With Atrial Fibrillation. Circ Cardiovasc Qual Outcomes. 2020;13(10):e006741

2. Schadendorf D, van den Bergh J, Verheij M, et al. Real-world safety and effectiveness of combined ipilimumab and nivolumab in advanced melanoma: the Dutch Melanoma Treatment Registry. Eur J Cancer. 2022;171:172–182.

3. Kakkar AK, Goldhaber SZ, Hull RD, et al. One-year outcomes after discharge for acute coronary syndrome in patients with atrial fibrillation: GARFIELD-AF. Eur Heart J Acute Cardiovasc Care. 2020;9(5):467–477.

4. Gupta S, Hayek SS, Wang W, et al. Factors Associated With Death in Critically Ill Patients With Coronavirus Disease 2019 in the US. JAMA Intern Med. 2020;180(11):1436–1447.

5. Klein NP, Lewis N, Goddard K, et al. Surveillance for Adverse Events After COVID-19 mRNA Vaccination. JAMA. 2021;326(14):1-10.

6. Wasserstein RL, Lazar NA. The ASA Statement on p-Values: Context, Process, and Purpose. Am Stat. 2016;70(2):129–133.

7. U.S. Food and Drug Administration. Real-World Data: Assessing Electronic Health Records and Medical Claims Data to Support Regulatory Decision-Making for Drug and Biological Products. Final Guidance for Industry. September 2024.

8. European Medicines Agency. Reflection paper on the use of real-world data in non interventional studies to generate real-world evidence for regulatory purposes. EMA/99865/2025. 2025.

9. International Council for Harmonisation. ICH M14 guideline on general principles on planning, designing, analysing, and reporting of non-interventional studies that utilise real-world data for safety assessment of medicines. Geneva: ICH; 2025.

10. International Council for Harmonisation. ICH E9(R1) addendum on estimands and sensitivity analysis in clinical trials to the guideline on statistical principles for clinical trials. Geneva: ICH; 2019.

11. Zheng SL, Roddick AJ. Association of Aspirin Use for Primary Prevention With Cardiovascular Events and Bleeding Events: A Systematic Review and Meta-analysis. JAMA. 2019;321(3):277-287.

12. Muller CJ, MacLehose RF. Estimating predicted probabilities from logistic regression: different methods correspond to different targets. Int J Epidemiol. 2014;43(3):962–970.

13. Uno H, Claggett B, Tian L, Inoue E, Gallo P, Miyata T, et al. Moving beyond the hazard ratio in quantifying the between-group difference in survival analysis. J Clin Oncol. 2014;32(22):2380–5.

14. Rumyantsev AA, Glazkova EV, Tikhomirova TE, et al. Frontline maintenance olaparib therapy for BRCA/HRD-positive

advanced epithelial ovarian cancer: real-world data analysis in matched population. BMC Med Res Methodol. 2013;13:152.

15. Dang A, Vallish BN, Dang A, et al. Use of real-world evidence to support FDA approval of oncology drugs. Value Health. 2020;23(10):1358–65.

16. DeMichele A, Cristofanilli M, Brufsky A, et al. Comparative effectiveness of first-line palbociclib plus letrozole versus letrozole alone for HR+/HER2− metastatic breast cancer in US real-world clinical practice. Breast Cancer Res. 2021;23(1):37.

17. Anker SD, Butler J, Filippatos G, , et al. Empagliflozin in heart failure with a preserved ejection fraction. N Engl J Med. 2021;385(16):1451–61.

18. Heerspink HJL, Karasik A, Thuresson M, et al. Kidney outcomes associated with use of SGLT2 inhibitors in real-world clinical practice (CVD-REAL 3): a multinational observational cohort study. Lancet Diabetes Endocrinol. 2020;8(1):27–35.

19. Richardson PG, Riches ML, Kernan NA, et al. Phase 3 trial of defibrotide for the treatment of severe veno-occlusive disease and multi-organ failure. Blood. 2016;127(13):1656–65.

20. Asano J, Sugano H, Murakami H, et al. PMDA perspective on use of real-world data and real-world evidence as an external control: recent examples and considerations. Clin Pharmacol Ther. 2025;117(4):910–9.

21. Nishioka K, Makimura T, Ishiguro A, et al. Evolving acceptance and use of RWE for regulatory decision making on the benefit/risk assessment of a drug in Japan. Clin Pharmacol Ther. 2022;111(1):35–43.

# Chapter 9. Reading and Critically Appraisal of a Study

Real-world evidence (RWE) studies are increasingly cited in clinical guidelines, regulatory submissions, reimbursement decisions, and health technology assessments. Yet unlike randomized controlled trials (RCTs), which follow well-standardized reporting conventions and methodological expectations, RWE studies encompass a wide spectrum of designs, data sources, and analytic strategies - each with distinct strengths and vulnerabilities. The absence of a universal "gold standard" for conducting RWE means that readers must rely on critical appraisal skills that go beyond superficial metrics (e.g., p-values or sample size) to assess the validity, transparency, and applicability of study findings.

This chapter equips readers with a pragmatic, stepwise framework to evaluate RWE studies efficiently and rigorously. Drawing on established tools (e.g., the ISPE–ISPOR checklist [1], GRACE principles [2], and the STROBE statement [3]), as well as recent regulatory guidance from the FDA [4], EMA [5], and the ICH M14 [6] guideline, which provides the first global harmonized framework for the design and analysis of RWE safety studies, we emphasize **what to look for** rather than **what to calculate**.

Each element of appraisal is illustrated with concrete examples from published literature - across therapeutic areas and geographies - to ground the discussion in real-world contexts. As in other chapters, we maintain a global perspective, referencing examples from the United States (e.g., Medicare claims analyses), Europe (e.g., EUnetHTA collaborations), and low- and middle-income settings (e.g., cancer registry studies in Latin America).

The structure of this chapter follows the natural workflow of a reader encountering an RWE study for the first time: starting with title and abstract screening, progressing through methodology, results, and interpretation, and concluding with synthesis and decision-making implications. At each step, we provide a distilled checklist, flag common methodological pitfalls, and illustrate how even a well-executed study can mislead if its assumptions or generalizability are overlooked.

## 9.1. A Practical Checklist

**Before delving into specific components,**

Table 9.1 presents a high-level, 10-item checklist distilled from major appraisal frameworks and adapted to reflect the realities of contemporary RWE publication (many of which lack full protocol registration or pre-specified analysis plans). This checklist is not a scoring tool; rather, it serves as a mental scaffolding to guide systematic interrogation of any RWE report.

This table can be reproduced on a single half-page as a quick-reference sidebar (e.g., inserted after the first major subsection). We recommend placing it after a brief narrative (see below) to avoid abrupt visual onset.

## 9.2. Red Flags: Common Warning Signs

Before examining methodological details, experienced readers scan for "red flags", features that, while not definitive proof of flawed science, warrant heightened scrutiny. These often arise from publication pressures, incomplete reporting, or misaligned incentives.

**Table 9.1 Core Questions for Critical Appraisal of an RWE Study**

| Domain | Key Question |
|---|---|
| **Research Question** | Is the question clearly defined, answerable with the chosen data, and relevant to a decision context (e.g., regulatory, clinical, policy)? |
| **Data Source(s)** | Are the source(s) described in sufficient detail - including provenance, structure, limitations, and validation status? Is a Common Data Model (CDM) (e.g., OMOP) used to ensure reproducibility? Are linkages documented? |
| **Population Definition** | Are inclusion/exclusion criteria reproducible? Are key baseline characteristics reported (e.g., age, sex, comorbidities, prior treatments)? |
| **Exposure & Outcome Definitions** | Are these operationalized objectively (e.g., drug dispensing vs. self-report)? Are coding systems (e.g., ICD-10, ATC) specified? |
| **Study Design** | Is the chosen design (cohort, case–control, etc.) appropriate for the question? If comparative, is the comparator group clinically meaningful? |
| **Confounding Control** | Are potential confounders identified a priori? Are methods (e.g., propensity scores, regression, instrumental variables) described and justified? Are sensitivity analyses presented? |
| **Missing Data & Measurement Error** | Is the extent and mechanism of missingness addressed? Are strategies for handling it (e.g., multiple imputation) stated? |
| **Statistical Analysis** | Are effect measures appropriate (e.g., hazard ratios for time-to-event)? Are confidence intervals reported? Is multiplicity addressed? |
| **Transparency & Reproducibility** | Is a protocol available (e.g., on ClinicalTrials.gov or HMA-EMA Catalogue or published e.g. in Annals of Real-World Data & Evidence)? Are analytic code or data dictionaries shared? |
| **Interpretation & Generalizability** | Do the authors distinguish statistical significance from clinical relevance? Are limitations contextualized? Are external validity boundaries acknowledged? |

A frequent red flag is outcome switching without justification: for example, a study registered to assess heart failure hospitalization as the primary endpoint suddenly reporting a composite of "CV events" in the published manuscript, with no rationale for the change.

A striking U.S.-based example involves a large population-based cohort study of SGLT2 inhibitors versus GLP-1 receptor agonists using Medicare and commercial claims data, in which initial prespecified analyses focused on hospitalization for heart failure were subsequently expanded post hoc to include a broader composite of cardiovascular outcomes -raising questions about whether the full comparative effectiveness picture was being presented selectively rather than systematically [7].

In Europe, the EMA's 2025 Reflection Paper on the use of real-world data in non-interventional studies explicitly requires that protocols be registered and pre-specified prior to study initiation, and that any deviations from the pre-specified analysis plan be scientifically justified - a requirement that applies particularly to post-authorisation safety studies (PASS) governed by GVP Module VIII [5].

Another red flag is **overreliance on statistical significance without clinical anchoring**. Readers should be wary when an adjusted hazard ratio of 0.92 (95% CI: 0.87–0.98) is heralded as "significant risk reduction," yet the absolute risk difference is <0.1% over 5 years - a finding unlikely to alter practice despite nominal significance. Conversely, a hazard ratio of 1.25 (95% CI: 0.98–1.58) may be dismissed as "non-significant," even if the point estimate suggests a potentially meaningful signal warranting further monitoring - especially in safety contexts.

A third and increasingly common red flag is **data provenance opacity**. With the proliferation of commercial real-world data (RWD) platforms (e.g., Flatiron, IQVIA, Cegedim), studies sometimes cite only the vendor name without describing data capture mechanisms, update frequency, or validation against gold standards. Real-world studies of biosimilar use in rheumatoid arthritis across Europe illustrate this risk concretely: multi-country analyses drawing on commercial claims databases have repeatedly been found to represent only a subset of European healthcare systems - often limited to countries where hospital-dispensed biologics are captured in claims - while silently excluding outpatient or homecare dispensing channels through which a substantial proportion of biologics are actually delivered in settings such as Germany and France. Without explicit disclosure of these structural gaps, claims of "European" representativeness are misleading [9].

Commercial platforms are not alone, and lack of transparency is also common among public or governmental platforms. The author had to withdraw a German Statutory Health Insurance Data from a large multi-country post authorization safety study (PASS) sponsored by pharmaceutical consortium, due to the platform refusal to be audited by a third party. They simply considered they were not to be audited as they were a public party!

## 9.3. Interpreting Results: Beyond the Point Estimate

Once methodological robustness has been assessed, the reader must interpret the results - not in isolation, but in relation to the clinical or policy question at hand. This requires distinguishing statistical from clinical and decision-relevant significance.

Consider a U.S. cohort study of direct oral anticoagulants (DOACs) versus warfarin in atrial fibrillation, using Optum's Clinformatics Data Mart [10]. The reported adjusted hazard ratio (aHR) for intracranial hemorrhage among apixaban versus warfarin was 0.24 (95% CI: 0.12–0.50, $p<0.001$), widely reported in the media as "76% lower risk." However, the absolute risk reduction was 0.77 events per 100 person-years - translating to a number needed to treat (NNT) of ~130 over one year to prevent one event. In a population where baseline bleeding risk is already low, this may not outweigh concerns about cost, monitoring burden, or patient preference. Another study using a Swedish cohort showed a higher absolute benefit due to older and more comorbid population [11].

**Effect modification** is another critical layer. An RWE study of pembrolizumab in advanced NSCLC using the nationwide French ESCKEYP cohort demonstrated that pooled survival estimates across all PD-L1 positive patients (TPS ≥1%) obscured substantial effect modification: outcomes in patients with TPS ≥50% were markedly more favourable than in those with TPS 1–49%, consistent with clinical trial data showing HRs approaching 0.50 in high expressors but near 1.0 in low expressors [12]. Without pre-specified stratification by TPS, clinicians risk overgeneralizing efficacy across the full PD-L1 positive population.

In safety studies, confidence intervals often convey more than point estimates. The Harmony Outcomes trial of albiglutide - a GLP-1 receptor agonist - reported a myocardial infarction hazard ratio of 0.96 (95% CI: 0.74 - 1.25) [13]. Although the point estimate was near null and the overall primary MACE endpoint showed benefit, the MI confidence interval was wide and crossed 1.0, illustrating how an individual component can remain genuinely uncertain even within an overall favorable safety profile - a reminder that inconclusive evidence for a specific outcome requires acknowledgement of remaining uncertainty rather than blanket reassurance.

Table 9.2 provides interpreting effects and questions to ask about effect measures in an RWE study report. Note that no single effect measure is universally "best" - the choice must align with the study design, outcome type, and decision context.

**Table 9.2 Interpreting Effect Measures in RWE and questions to ask.**

| Measure | Typical Use Case | What to Ask |
|---|---|---|
| **Risk Ratio (RR)** | Cumulative incidence over fixed follow-up (e.g., 1-year MACE) | Is follow-up sufficiently complete? Is loss to follow-up differential? |
| **Odds Ratio (OR)** | Case–control or cross-sectional studies | Is the outcome rare (<10%)? If not, OR may overstate RR. |
| **Hazard Ratio (HR)** | Time-to-event (e.g., hospitalization, death) | Are proportional hazards assumptions tested? Is censoring informative? |
| **Rate Ratio (IRR)** | Recurrent events (e.g., asthma exacerbations) | Is the person-time denominator accurately captured? |
| **Absolute Risk Difference (ARD)** | Benefit–risk communication | Is the baseline risk specified? Is the time horizon clinically meaningful? |

## 9.4. Synthesizing Appraisal into Actionable Judgment

Critical appraisal does not end with identifying flaws; it culminates in a reasoned judgment about whether - and how - the study should inform decisions. This synthesis requires weighing methodological rigor against pragmatic utility.

For regulatory and reimbursement decisions, FDA and EMA, and progressively other regulators and health technology bodies emphasize that no single RWE study is definitive. Rather, evidence is evaluated as part of a "totality" argument - where consistency across studies, biological plausibility, and alignment with RCT data (if available) matter more than any isolated p-value. For example, the original 2016 FDA approval of nusinersen for SMA drew on multiple complementary studies - including the Phase 3 ENDEAR trial in symptomatic infants and the NURTURE study in presymptomatic infants - alongside emerging registry data from the SMArtCARE registry in Europe. No single dataset was definitive in isolation, but their coherence across designs and populations formed the regulatory basis for approval, illustrating how diverse evidence streams can collectively support a decision when each provides a piece of the clinical puzzle [14, 15].

For clinical guidelines, committees such as NICE (UK) or HAS (France) apply GRADE-adapted criteria for RWE [16]. A 2019 French equivalence study using the national SNDS healthcare database compared biosimilar (CT-P13) and reference infliximab in 5,050 infliximab-naïve patients with Crohn's disease, demonstrating equivalent composite outcomes within a pre-specified 10% non-inferiority margin - without randomization and with a follow-up limited to approximately 2.5 years [17]. HAS considered this evidence in its reassessments of infliximab biosimilar reimbursement, weighting it alongside NOR-SWITCH trial data, explicitly because it filled a critical evidence gap - long-term real-world effectiveness in the broader, more heterogeneous IBD population not captured by RCTs conducted primarily in rheumatology settings.

For hospital or health system decisions, pragmatic considerations dominate: Is the population comparable to ours? Can we replicate the exposure? Is the outcome measurable in our EHR? The EGDT experience illustrates this vividly. The original Rivers trial reported a 16% absolute mortality reduction in septic shock patients at a single urban U.S. emergency department - a result widely adopted into international guidelines. Yet when three large multicenter trials (ProCESS, ARISE, ProMISe) replicated the protocol across U.S., Australian, and UK ICUs, no mortality benefit was found [18]. The PRISM individual-patient meta-analysis confirmed that usual care in 2014 already incorporated most EGDT principles, leaving no treatment gap to close [19] - a reminder that the local care environment determines whether implementing a published protocol adds value or merely formalizes existing practice.

## 9.5. Educational Material and Applied Tools

Critical appraisal is most useful when it produces a structured output that is legible to the decision-maker who commissioned it - whether a clinician selecting a treatment protocol, a guideline committee weighing evidence, or a formulary board evaluating a new biosimilar. Box 9.1 provides a reporting template that adapts the appraisal scope and language to the relevant stakeholder, translating the ten-item checklist in Table 9.1 into actionable conclusions rather than methodological verdicts. The goal is to provide overall confidence about the evidence and determine how it can be used in decision making.

Readers wishing to apply these principles interactively can check the accompanying **EvidenceMastery™** website which QR code is provided at the beginning of this book. Aside from the additional learning material, they can also try **AppraiseAi™** developed by the author to provide a critical appraisal of a manuscript using artificial intelligence. Users can upload a manuscript and observe how the system applies each appraisal domain - study design, confounding, data provenance, effect measure interpretation - producing a structured appraisal in real time. The tool does not replace expert judgment, but it makes the appraisal process transparent and reproducible, helping readers internalize the reasoning steps described throughout this chapter.

**Box 9.1 RWE Critical Appraisal Summary Sheet**

**Study ID**: [Author, Year, Journal]
**Decision Context**:
☐ Regulatory ☐ Reimbursement ☐ Clinical Guideline ☐ Operational

**1. Question & Relevance**
Clear, answerable question? ☐ Yes ☐ Partial ☐ No
Aligns with decision need? ☐ Strong ☐ Moderate ☐ Weak
**2. Data Fitness-for-Purpose**
Source(s):
Key limitations (e.g., coding lag, no lab values)?
Linkage documented? ☐ Yes ☐ No
**3. Design & Comparability**
Design: ☐ Cohort ☐ Case–control ☐ Cross-sectional ☐ Hybrid
Comparator: ☐ Active treatment ☐ Placebo/no treatment ☐ Historical
Clinically plausible? ☐ Yes ☐ Unclear
**4. Bias & Confounding**
Key confounders measured? ☐ All major ☐ Some ☐ Few
Method used: ____________________________
Sensitivity analyses? ☐ Yes (describe: ______) ☐ No
5. **Results Interpretation**
Effect measure: _______ (e.g., aHR = __)
Absolute benefit/harm: __________
CI includes null? ☐ Yes ☐ No
Clinical relevance: ☐ High ☐ Moderate ☐ Low
**6. Overall Confidence**
☐ High (suitable as primary evidence)
☐ Moderate (supportive, needs corroboration)
☐ Low (hypothesis-generating only)

**Comments**: ____________________________________

## 9.6. Conclusion

Reading and appraising RWE studies is not a mechanical checklist exercise; it is a disciplined form of scientific skepticism married to pragmatic judgment. The explosion of RWD sources and analytic tools has democratized evidence generation - but also amplified the risk of misleading conclusions from poorly designed or inadequately reported studies. Mastery of critical appraisal enables clinicians, regulators, and health economists to separate signal from noise, to recognize when an RWE study adds to the evidence base - and when it merely adds "volume".

As RWE becomes embedded in routine decision-making, the onus is on readers to ask not only what the study found, but how confidently and for whom. A well-appraised RWE study may not meet the internal validity bar of an RCT - but when its limitations are transparent, its assumptions are defensible, and its context aligned, it can offer insights no RCT ever could: about long-term outcomes, rare events, diverse populations, and the messy reality of everyday care.

## References

1. Berger ML, Sox H, Willke RJ, et al. Good practices for real-world data studies of treatment and/or comparative effectiveness: recommendations from the Joint ISPOR–ISPE Special Task Force on Real-World Evidence in Health Care Decision Making. Value Health. 2017;20(8):1003–8.

2. Dreyer NA, Bryant A, Velentgas P. The GRACE Checklist: A Validated Assessment Tool for High Quality Observational Studies of Comparative Effectiveness. J Manag Care Spec Pharm. 2016;22(10):1107-13.

3. von Elm E, Altman DG, Egger M, et al. The Strengthening the Reporting of Observational Studies in Epidemiology (STROBE) statement: guidelines for reporting observational studies. J Clin Epidemiol. 2007;60(10):1073–1081.

4. U.S. Food and Drug Administration. Framework for FDA's Real-World Evidence Program. December 2018.

5. European Medicines Agency. Reflection paper on the use of real-world data in non-interventional studies to generate real-world evidence for regulatory purposes. EMA/99865/2025. 2025.

6. International Council for Harmonisation. ICH M14 guideline on general principles on planning, designing, analysing, and reporting of

non-interventional studies that utilise real-world data for safety assessment of medicines. Geneva: ICH; 2024.

7. Patorno E, Htoo PT, Glynn RJ, et al. Sodium–Glucose Cotransporter-2 Inhibitors Versus Glucagon-like Peptide-1 Receptor Agonists and the Risk for Cardiovascular Outcomes in Routine Care Patients With Diabetes Across Categories of Cardiovascular Disease. Ann Intern Med. 2021;174(11):1528–41..

8. an Hylckama Vlieg A, Helmerhorst FM, Vandenbroucke JP, Doggen CJM, Rosendaal FR. The venous thrombotic risk of oral contraceptives, effects of oestrogen dose and progestogen type: results of the MEGA case-control study. BMJ. 2009;339:b2921.

9. Michaud K, Wolfe F. Comparative effectiveness research for biologic therapies in inflammatory arthritis: Challenges and opportunities in the real-world evidence setting. Clin Exp Rheumatol. 2021;39 Suppl 134(6):41–50.

10. Yao X, Abraham NS, Sangaralingham LR, et al. Effectiveness and Safety of Dabigatran, Rivaroxaban, and Apixaban Versus Warfarin in Nonvalvular Atrial Fibrillation. J Am Heart Assoc. 2016;5(6):e003725.

11. Rutherford OW, Jonasson C, Ghanima W, Söderdahl F, Halvorsen S. Effectiveness and safety of oral anticoagulants in elderly patients with atrial fibrillation. Heart. 2022;108(5):345–52.

12. Descourt R, Greillier L, Perol M, et al. First-line single-agent pembrolizumab for PD-L1-positive (tumor proportion score ≥50%) advanced non-small cell lung cancer in the real world: impact in brain metastasis: a national French multicentric cohort (ESCKEYP GFPC study). Cancer Immunol Immunother. 2023;72(1):91–9.

13. Hernandez AF, Green JB, Janmohamed S, et al; Harmony Outcomes Committees and Investigators. Albiglutide and cardiovascular outcomes in patients with type 2 diabetes and cardiovascular disease (Harmony Outcomes): a double-blind, randomised placebo-controlled trial. Lancet. 2018;392(10157):1519–29.

14. Finkel RS, Mercuri E, Darras BT, Connolly AM, Kuntz NL, Kirschner J, et al; ENDEAR Study Group. Nusinersen versus Sham

Control in Infantile-Onset Spinal Muscular Atrophy. N Engl J Med. 2017;377(18):1723–32.

15. De Vivo DC, Bertini E, Swoboda KJ, et al. Nusinersen initiated in infants during the presymptomatic stage of spinal muscular atrophy: interim efficacy and safety results from the Phase 2 NURTURE study. Neuromuscul Disord. 2019;29(11):842–56.

16. Schünemann HJ, Cuello C, Akl EA, et al; GRADE Working Group. GRADE guidelines: 18. How ROBINS-I and other tools to assess risk of bias in nonrandomized studies should be used to rate the certainty of a body of evidence. J Clin Epidemiol. 2019;111:105–14.

17. Meyer A, Rudant J, Drouin J, et al. Effectiveness and safety of reference infliximab and biosimilar in Crohn disease: a French equivalence study. Ann Intern Med. 2019;170(2):99–107.

18. PRISM Investigators; Rowan KM, Angus DC, Bailey M, et al. Early, goal-directed therapy for septic shock - a patient-level meta-analysis. N Engl J Med. 2017;376(23):2223–34.

19. Yealy DM, Kellum JA, Huang DT, et al; ProCESS Investigators. A randomized trial of protocol-based care for early septic shock. N Engl J Med. 2014;370(18):1683–93.

# Part III: Real-World Evidence in Practice

# Chapter 10. RWE in Regulatory Decision-Making

Regulatory decision-making has traditionally relied on randomized controlled trials (RCTs) to establish the safety and efficacy of medical products. However, as healthcare systems demand more timely, generalizable, and context-specific evidence, regulators have increasingly incorporated real-world evidence (RWE) into their evaluation frameworks.

The shift reflects a recognition that RWE can complement, extend, or - under certain rigorous conditions - substitute for RCT data, particularly in post-marketing phases or for rare diseases where RCTs are impractical. In this chapter, we examine how key regulatory authorities - namely the U.S. Food and Drug Administration (FDA), the European Medicines Agency (EMA), and the UK Medicines and Healthcare products Regulatory Agency (MHRA) - have evolved their policies and practices for evaluating RWE. We highlight landmark submissions, methodological expectations, and emerging harmonization efforts. Throughout, we emphasize the importance of study design robustness, transparency, and relevance to the regulatory question at hand.

## 10.1. The Regulatory Landscape

Over the past decade, regulatory agencies have moved from exploratory pilot programs to formal guidance and operational frameworks for RWE. This evolution has been driven not only by advances in data infrastructure (e.g., national electronic health record networks, large claims databases) but also by legislative mandates and stakeholder consensus.

In the United States, the 21st Century Cures Act (2016) explicitly tasked the FDA with developing a framework to evaluate RWE for new indications or post-approval study requirements [1]. In Europe, the Clinical Trials Regulation (EU No 536/2014) and the EU Pharmaceutical Strategy (2020) underscored the need for innovative evidence streams, including RWE, to support regulatory decision-making across the product lifecycle [2]. The United Kingdom, post-Brexit, has pursued an agile, innovation-friendly approach through the MHRA's Innovative Licensing and Access Pathway (ILAP) and its 2022 RWE strategy [3].

While motivations differ - expediting access in the U.S., enhancing sustainability in Europe, and positioning the UK as a regulatory science leader - the underlying expectation remains consistent: RWE must be fit for purpose. A study's fitness is judged not just by the volume or novelty of the data, but by how well the design, analysis plan, and data provenance align with the specific regulatory question (e.g., safety signal detection vs. comparative effectiveness for label expansion).

## 10.2. U.S. FDA

The FDA's embrace of RWE is anchored in four key documents:

1. **The Framework for Real-World Evidence** (2018): Outlined four priority use cases: (i) generating external control arms, (ii) supplementing RCT evidence for rare diseases, (iii) supporting label expansions, and (iv) post-marketing safety monitoring [4].

2. **RWE Guidance for Industry** (2021): Provided detailed methodological expectations for RWE submissions supporting new indications of already approved drugs [5].
3. **Project Orbis RWE Pilot** (2022): A multinational initiative (with Australia, Canada, Singapore, and Switzerland) to evaluate RWE submissions in parallel across agencies, signaling convergence in standards [6].
4. **Data Standards for RWE Submissions** (2024): The FDA finalized its guidance on the use of electronic health records and medical claims data, emphasizing the requirement for data to be submitted in a format the FDA can process, such as CDISC SDTM, which remains a hurdle for many RWD sources [7].

## 10.2.1. Regulatory Acceptance Criteria

For an RWE study to be considered in a regulatory submission, the FDA expects:

- **A pre-specified analytic plan:** including primary/secondary endpoints, covariates, and statistical methods, ideally registered in a public repository.
- **Evidence of data fitness:** documentation of data provenance, coding standards (e.g., SNOMED-CT, LOINC in EHRs), and validation of key variables.
- **Transparent handling of confounding**: e.g., via propensity score matching, instrumental variable analysis, or target trial emulation.
- **Sensitivity analyses**: to assess robustness of conclusions.

## 10.2.2. Notable FDA Approvals Supported by RWE

**Label expansion for tacrolimus for lung transplantation**

In 2021, the FDA approved a supplemental indication for tacrolimus for the prevention of organ rejection in adult and pediatric lung transplant recipients - making it the first immunosuppressant ever approved for this population. Crucially, the sNDA was supported not by a randomized trial but by a pre-specified, non-interventional retrospective cohort study using data from the U.S. Scientific Registry of Transplant Recipients (SRTR), a federally mandated database capturing all organ transplant procedures in the United States. The RWE study enrolled 25,355 adult deceased-donor lung transplant recipients between 1999 and 2017, with mortality ascertained through linkage to the Social Security Administration Death Master File. One-year graft survival in tacrolimus-based regimens reached approximately 91% in adults and 92% in pediatric recipients, compared with a well-documented natural history of early graft failure in the absence of effective immunosuppression - an effect magnitude sufficiently large that confounding could not plausibly explain the observed benefit. The FDA formally determined that this non-interventional study, compared against these historical controls, met statutory requirements for an "adequate and well-controlled study" under 21 CFR 314.126. FDA reviewers highlighted this approval as a landmark illustration that fit-for-purpose RWD drawn from a comprehensive national registry - when the effect size is large, the data source covers the full target population, and the analytical plan is pre-specified - can independently satisfy evidentiary standards for confirmatory effectiveness claims, rather than serving merely as supplementary or contextualizing evidence [8, 9].

**Fosdenopterin approval with RWE as external control**

In 2021, the FDA approved fosdenopterin to reduce mortality risk in patients with molybdenum cofactor deficiency (MoCD) Type A - a fatal ultra-rare inborn error of metabolism with an estimated US prevalence of approximately 50 patients. Conducting a randomized trial was ethically and numerically impossible: the disease causes death in most patients within the first years of life, with a median survival of 36 months without treatment. The sNDA therefore rested on three single-arm clinical studies (n=13 treated patients) compared against 18 genotype-matched, untreated patients from a prospectively constructed natural history registry, the ALX-MCD-502 study. Efficacy was assessed as overall survival at three years: 84% in treated patients versus 55% in historical controls, representing an 82% reduction in the risk of death. The FDA accepted this RWE-based external control arm as meeting the "substantial evidence of effectiveness" standard, noting that the well-characterized, uniformly lethal natural history of MoCD Type A - and the use of genotype matching to minimize selection bias - mitigated the principal confounding concerns of non-randomized historical comparisons. This approval exemplifies the regulatory role of rigorously assembled natural history data in ultra-rare diseases where prospective randomized evidence is unattainable [10].

## 10.3. European Medicines Agency (EMA)

Unlike the FDA, the EMA does not have direct authority over national health systems and thus relies heavily on collaboration with member states and methodological networks - most notably the Innovative Medicines Initiative (IMI) projects (e.g., EMIF, EHDEN) and the EU-ADR network [11,12]. The sponsorship of the European Network of Centres for Phamracoepidemiology and Pharmacovigilance (ENCePP) [13] gives EMA a significant headway in shaping the practice of RWE.

Key milestones include:

1. **EMA conceptual framework for RWE (2019):** EMA staff outlined the need for fit-for-purpose RWD and distinguished between exploratory (hypothesis-generating) and confirmatory (hypothesis-testing) uses of RWE across the product lifecycle, noting that RWD acceptance for efficacy/effectiveness claims required substantially higher evidentiary standards than for safety surveillance [14].
2. **Revised Guideline on Good Pharmacovigilance Practices (GVP Module VIII, 2017)**: Formalized expectations for using RWE in post-authorization safety studies (PASS) [15].
3. **EMA Big Data Steering Group (2020–2024):** Coordinated cross-divisional RWE review and advised on methodological standards including the Data Quality Framework for EU medicines regulation and the development of DARWIN EU [16].

4. **EMA Reflection Paper (2024)**: The EMA finalized its "Reflection paper on real-world evidence in support of regulatory decision-making," providing a roadmap for the use of RWE across the product lifecycle, from pre-authorization to post-marketing [17].

### 10.3.1. Notable EMA Approvals Supported by RWE

**Fostamatinib for immune thrombocytopenia (ITP)**

In 2020, the EMA authorized fostamatinib for ITP in adults refractory to previous treatment, based on two phase 3 placebo-controlled trials. The Committee for Human Medicinal Products (CHMP) noted that the available RCT data lacked sufficient precision in subgroups such as older adults and patients with cardiovascular comorbidities, and required post-authorization data collection to address these uncertainties - illustrating how regulators may use RWE planning as a condition of approval when trial populations are narrow [18]. The RWE matched the RCT's inclusion/exclusion criteria as closely as possible, using time-varying exposure definitions and inverse probability weighting to emulate randomization.

**Alglucosidase alfa with RWE as external control**

Alglucosidase alfa received European Commission marketing authorization in 2006 as the first treatment for Pompe disease, a rare, rapidly fatal lysosomal storage disorder. For infantile-onset disease, a prospective randomized controlled trial was ethically and practically impossible: untreated infants uniformly die of cardiorespiratory failure before the age of one year. The CHMP therefore accepted a single-arm open-label study (n=18 infants aged <6 months) in which efficacy was assessed against an untreated natural history historical control group (n=42 patients). All 18 treated infants were alive at 18 months of age, and 15 remained ventilator-free; in contrast, only 1 of the 42 historical controls survived to 18 months. The CHMP explicitly endorsed this natural history comparator as the primary evidence basis, concluding that an effect of this magnitude could not be explained by confounding. This case established a foundational precedent in EU regulatory science: that real-world natural history data can constitute adequate comparative evidence for marketing authorization when the effect size is large and randomization is infeasible.

### 10.3.2. Data Sources and Quality Expectations

As shown in Table 10.1, EMA reviewers expect RWE submissions to include a data quality assessment report, expecting documentation in the domains such as completeness, accuracy, consistency and representativeness of the data. The fitness for use (purpose) is at the center of the appraisal of any data source fir any given goal.

**Table 10.1 EMA-Recommended Domains for RWE Data Quality Assessment**

| Domain | Expected Documentation |
|---|---|
| **Completeness** | % missing for key variables (e.g., lab values, concomitant medications); strategies for handling missingness |
| **Accuracy** | Validation studies (e.g., chart review vs. EHR entry for diagnosis codes); positive predictive values (PPV) for key endpoints |
| **Consistency** | Temporal plausibility (e.g., drug start before lab test); cross-source concordance (e.g., hospital discharge codes vs. claims); logical consistency (e.g., prostate cancer vs. gender) |
| **Representativeness** | Comparison of study cohort demographics vs. national epidemiology (e.g., cancer incidence by age/sex) |

## 10.4. UK MHRA

The MHRA has positioned RWE at the core of its post-Brexit regulatory strategy, emphasizing speed without compromising scientific rigor. Its **Real World Evidence Framework** articulates three strategic objectives: (i) enable earlier patient access, (ii) support life-cycle management, and (iii) strengthen pharmacovigilance [3].

**Key Initiatives**

- **Innovative Licensing and Access Pathway (ILAP)**: Integrates RWE planning early via the Target Development

Profile (TDP), where sponsors specify how RWE will address evidence gaps across development phases.

- **MHRA RWE Scientific Dialogue Programme:** During the pilot four applicants were selected for closed-door, confidential meetings with the MHRA and one for the pre-competitive, 'safe harbour', workshop jointly convened by the MHRA and the National Institute for Health and Care Excellence (NICE).
- **Collaboration with NHS Digital & OpenSAFELY**: Leverages England's unified primary care database (covering >57 million patients) for rapid signal detection and effectiveness studies [19].

## 10.4.1. Notable MHRA approval supported by RWE

**Fluticasone Furoate/Vilanterol for COPD and Asthma**

The Salford Lung Study (SLS) was the world's first phase III pragmatic randomized controlled trial of a pre-licensed medicine conducted entirely in routine clinical practice, using linked electronic health records as the sole data source. In the COPD arm, 2,799 patients from 75 general practices were randomized 1:1 to once-daily fluticasone furoate/vilanterol (FF/VI 100/25 μg) or usual care over 12 months. FF/VI produced a statistically significant 8.4% relative reduction in moderate-to-severe exacerbations versus usual care (rate ratio 0.92; 95% CI 0.85–0.99; p=0.025), with no significant difference in serious adverse events or pneumonia. The asthma arm (n=4,233) similarly demonstrated superior asthma control as measured by the Asthma Control Test at 52 weeks (OR 1.75; 95% CI 1.55–1.98; p<0.0001). The MHRA, in joint scientific advice with NICE, approved the study design prospectively - a regulatory first - establishing that phase III effectiveness evidence generated through EHR-based pragmatic trials could satisfy UK regulatory standards [20, 21].

# 10.5. Comparative Insights: FDA vs. EMA vs. MHRA

While all three agencies prioritize methodological rigor, differences in governance and healthcare structure drive nuanced expectations. Table 10.2 provides a comparison of key RWE focuses of the regulators.

**Table 10.2 Regulatory Agency Comparison on Key RWE aspects**

| Aspect | FDA | EMA | MHRA |
|---|---|---|---|
| **Primary data sources for submissions** | U.S. claims (e.g., Medicare, Optum), oncology EHRs (Flatiron, COTA) | Multi-country registries (e.g., SWEDEHEART), national health databases (e.g., CPRD, SNDS), networks (e.g., EHDEN) | NHS primary/secondary care data (OpenSAFELY, HES, CPRD), UK Biobank linkage |
| **Pre-submission engagement** | Type C meetings, INTERACT program (early feasibility) | Scientific Advice Procedure (SAP), parallel EMA–HTA advice | ILAP Target Development Profile (TDP) with embedded RWE plan |
| **Acceptance of single-arm RWE for efficacy** | Rare in confirmatory settings; limited to rare/orphan diseases or as external controls | Generally requires comparator; accepts single-arm only for safety/signal generation | Open to single-arm in pandemic/emergency contexts if bias is rigorously mitigated |
| **Transparency expectations** | Analytic code (e.g., SAS, R) submission optional but encouraged | Code sharing encouraged via HMA-EMA Catalogue; Prtotocol registration mandatory for PASS | Full reproducibility package (code, synthetic data, analysis environment) expected for priority submissions |

## 10.6. Global Perspectives

### 10.6.1. Japan (PMDA)

PMDA has progressively expanded its use of RWE through MID-NET, a real-world database network linking electronic medical records and claims data across 23 partner hospitals. PMDA has accepted RWD/RWE as external controls in new drug applications primarily for orphan diseases, where RCT feasibility is limited. PMDA established a formal RWD Working Group in April 2021 to systematize methodological standards and regulatory guidance for RWE submissions across the product lifecycle [22].

### 10.6.2. Australia (TGA)

The Therapeutic Goods Administration (TGA) formally reviewed its use of RWE in 2021 and has since adopted FDA and EMA international scientific guidelines on RWD/RWE to harmonize its evidence requirements with comparable overseas regulators. The TGA accepts pragmatic trials, external-control studies, registry data, and observational studies for both premarket and post-market decisions, assessed case-by-case against standards of data relevance and reliability. A landmark example is the Australian Orthopaedic Association National Joint Replacement Registry (AOANJRR), whose real-time revision-rate data prompted the TGA to withdraw the DePuy ASR metal-on-metal hip implant from the Australian market in 2009 - nearly a year before the global recall [23,24].

### 10.6.3. Low- and Middle-Income Countries (LMICs)

In settings with fragmented data infrastructure, regulators are piloting pragmatic approaches:

- **The South African Health Products Regulatory Authority (SAHPRA)** has used real-world post-marketing data most visibly in the context of COVID-19 vaccine safety surveillance. Following the national vaccine rollout from May 2021, SAHPRA and the National Department of Health undertook disproportionality analysis of AEFI data across

37.5 million doses of BNT162b2 and Ad26.COV2.S vaccines administered between May 2021 and December 2022, detecting safety signals that informed regulatory communications and decisions. [25].

- **India's Central Drugs Standard Control Organisation (CDSCO)** has progressively integrated RWE approaches into its regulatory framework. In 2024, CDSCO waived the requirement for local clinical trials for drugs and vaccines already approved by stringent regulatory agencies - including the US FDA, EMA, MHRA, PMDA and TGA - in five categories including orphan drugs, gene and cellular therapies, and pandemic-related medicines. This policy treats foreign clinical and post-marketing evidence as sufficient for Indian approval, accelerating access while relying on externally generated RWE rather than mandating de novo local trials [26].

None of them does not yet have a formal standalone RWE guidance document equivalent to the FDA framework or EMA reflection paper. Their RWE use is primarily expressed through a **reliance model** (accepting foreign regulatory decisions as substitute evidence) and post-marketing pharmacovigilance, rather than through proactive RWE study generation for pre-approval decisions.

## 10.6.4. Harmonization of Methodological Expectations

Harmonization is accelerating through the ICH E9(R1) addendum on estimands [27] and the ICH M14 guideline on 'General Principles on Planning, Designing, Analysing and Reporting of Non-interventional Studies that Utilise Real-World Data' [28], complemented by the ICH Reflection Paper on pursuing harmonization of RWD/RWE for effectiveness evaluation [29]. Together, they lay the groundwork for the harmonization of methodological expectations:

1. **Estimand Alignment**

The study articulates the target trial it seeks to emulate - including population, treatment strategy, endpoint, and handling of intercurrent events - per ICH E9(R1).

2. **Robust Confounding Control**

   Passive adjustment (e.g., regression with covariates) is insufficient.

   Preferred methods include:

   - Propensity score matching/weighting with diagnostics (e.g., standardized mean differences <0.1)
   - Target trial emulation with time-varying exposures
   - Instrumental variable analysis (where valid instruments exist)
   - Sensitivity analyses using E-values or bias-analysis models

3. **Data Provenance & Validation**

   Sponsors must provide:

   - Data dictionary (coding systems, update frequency)
   - Validation metrics (PPV/NPV for key endpoints)
   - Documentation of data linkage methodology (e.g., deterministic vs. probabilistic), including error rates
   - Reproducibility Infrastructure

4. **Analytical transparency**

   While not yet mandatory everywhere, reviewers increasingly expect:

   - Version-controlled analytic code (e.g., GitHub repository)
   - Containerized execution environment (e.g., Dockerfile)

- o Synthetic or anonymized dataset for external replication
- o Sensitivity & Subgroup Analyses
- o Pre-specified sensitivity analyses (e.g., varying exposure definitions, unmeasured confounding scenarios) and effect modification assessment (e.g., age, comorbidity burden, care setting) are viewed as markers of thoroughness.

# 10.7. Emerging Trends and Challenges

As regulatory frameworks for real-world evidence mature, the field is entering a phase of accelerated innovation in both application and methodology. Sponsors, regulators, and health systems are collectively testing the boundaries of what RWE can credibly support - from replacing certain arms of traditional trials to enabling dynamic, near-real-time benefit–risk assessments. Yet with innovation comes complexity: novel designs such as **synthetic control arms** and **AI-augmented analytics** introduce new methodological considerations, while cross-border data governance and reproducibility remain persistent operational hurdles.

The trends emerging today reflect not just technological advancement, but a deeper reengineering of the evidence ecosystem itself - one that demands stronger alignment between scientific rigor, regulatory pragmatism, and ethical data stewardship.

## 10.7.1. Trend 1: The emergence of regulatory-supported RWD networks

The 2000s witnessed the birth of large-scale healthcare databases; the 2010s saw the maturation of pharmacoepidemiological methods to extract evidence from them. The current decade is defined by something qualitatively different: the emergence of federated data networks, cross-jurisdictional linkage infrastructure, and regulator-led data initiatives that connect previously siloed sources into actionable evidence ecosystems. Where earlier generations asked "can we collect the data?" and then "can we analyze it rigorously?", the 2020s are asking "can we connect it - securely, reproducibly, and at scale?" Box 10.1 provides a snapshot of the major RWD infrastructure initiatives in which regulators are active participants.

**Box 10.1 Global RWE Initiatives Snapshot (2023–2025)**

- **FDA Sentinel Initiative**: >300 million U.S. patient records for active safety surveillance; supports self-controlled case series and cohort studies.
- **EMA DARWIN EU**: As of 2024, DARWIN EU became fully operational, completing over 100 regulatory studies annually. It acts as a federated network across Europe, allowing the EMA and national regulators to execute rapid RWE studies without moving patient-level data.
- **NHS England OpenSAFELY**: Secure analytics platform providing query capabilities of primary care data (using herQL/common codes); with >50 peer-reviewed studies published (e.g., on anticoagulants, vaccines).
- **IMI EHDEN**: Provides a federated data network across 20+ European countries; offers open-source tools (e.g., OHDSI/OMOP) for standardized analysis.
- **OHDSI Global Network**: Over 100 data partners worldwide; promotes "one protocol, many analyses" reproducibility model.
- **WHO RWE Taskforce (2024 launch)**: Developing minimum standards for RWE in global health emergencies (e.g., antimicrobial resistance, pandemic therapeutics).

## 10.7.2. Trend 2: RWE in Accelerated Approval and Confirmatory Requirements

The FDA's recent policy shift allows sponsors to propose RWE-based post-marketing requirements (PMRs) to verify clinical benefit after accelerated approval - e.g., using EHR data to assess overall survival in oncology. However, this introduces tension: RWE studies may suffer from longer follow-up latency and attrition compared to prospective trials.

### 10.7.3. Trend 3: Regulatory Acceptance of Synthetic Control Arms

Synthetic control arms (SCAs), constructed from historical or external real-world data rather than randomizing patients to a control condition provide a methodological response to settings where placebo-controlled trials are ethically impractical or operationally infeasible. Once regarded with deep regulatory skepticism, SCAs have moved from the margins of evidence generation to a conditionally accepted tool at both FDA and EMA, particularly in rare diseases, oncology, and pediatrics. The question has shifted from "can observational data substitute for randomization?" to "under what conditions, with what causal inference methods, and with what pre-specification standards is it acceptable?".

### 10.7.4. Persistent Methodological and Governance Challenges

Despite the rapid institutionalization of RWE across regulatory frameworks, a set of structural challenges continues to constrain its consistent and reliable use in regulatory decision-making. These challenges are not merely technical - they reflect deeper tensions between the global ambition of RWE research and the fragmented legal, institutional, and scientific landscape within which it operates. Two of the most consequential are data governance and cross-border data transfer restrictions, which limit the feasibility of global studies, and the systematic underreporting of negative or null RWE findings, which distorts the evidence base available to regulators and prescribers alike.

- **Challenge 1: Data Governance and Cross-Border Transfers**

  GDPR (EU), HIPAA (U.S.), and emerging national data laws (e.g., Brazil's LGPD, India's DPDP Act) complicate multinational RWE studies. Federated analysis (e.g., via DataSHIELD or OHDSI's ARACHNE platform) is gaining traction: data remain local; only aggregated statistics or model parameters are shared. Furthermore, AI tools which transfer the data 'ghost' rather than the data are emerging, and then reconstitute the data once transferred are being suggested. But their validity and legality are yet to be verified.

- **Challenge 2: Publication Bias and Negative RWE**

  Unlike RCTs, negative RWE studies (e.g., failed label expansions) are rarely published, impeding learning. The author had a direct experience with this challenge while writing this book. The RWE Transparency Registry (proposed by ISPOR in 2024) seeks to address this by requiring protocol registration for all regulatory-intended RWE studies, regardless of outcome.

## 10.8. Conclusion

Regulatory acceptance of real-world evidence for drug approvals has matured from cautious exploration to structured integration - but it remains conditional. The FDA, EMA, and MHRA each articulate clear expectations: RWE must be fit for purpose, methodologically rigorous, and transparently reported. Landmark approvals demonstrate that high-quality RWE can influence labeling, safety monitoring, and access decisions, particularly when RCT evidence is incomplete or ungeneralizable. However, persistent challenges - data fragmentation, confounding, reproducibility, and legal heterogeneity - call for sustained collaboration between regulators, industry, academia, and health systems.

Looking ahead, harmonization through ICH, expansion of federated analytics, and the rise of AI-enabled bias diagnostics (e.g., causal machine learning for residual confounding) will shape the next generation of regulatory RWE. For sponsors, success hinges not on data volume alone, but on evidence architecture: aligning the regulatory question, data strategy, and analytical plan from the earliest development stages. In doing so, RWE evolves from a supplementary tool into a foundational pillar of evidence-based health regulation.

### References

1. 21st Century Cures Act, Public Law 114-255, 2016.

2. European Commission. Pharmaceutical Strategy for Europe. COM(2020) 761 final. Brussels: European Commission; 2020.

3. MHRA. Real World Evidence Framework. 2022.

4. FDA. Framework for Real-World Evidence Program. 2018.

5. FDA. Real-World Evidence: Assessing Electronic Health Records and Medical Claims Data to Support Regulatory Decision-Making for Drug and Biological Products. Guidance for Industry. 2021.

6. FDA. Project Orbis: Real-World Evidence Pilot. 2022.

7. FDA. Data Standards for Drug and Biological Product Submissions Containing Real-World Data. Guidance for Industry. 2024.

8. FDA. FDA approves new use of transplant drug based on real-world evidence [Press Release]. Silver Spring, MD: U.S. Food and Drug Administration; 2021 Jul 16.

9. Erdman J, Wolfram J, Nimke D, et al. Lung transplant outcomes in adults in the United States: retrospective cohort study using real-world evidence from the SRTR. Transplantation. 2022;106(6):1233–1242.

10. Farrell S, Karp J, Hager R, et al. Regulatory news: Nulibry (fosdenopterin) approved to reduce the risk of mortality in patients with molybdenum cofactor deficiency type A: FDA approval summary. J Inherit Metab Dis. 2021;44(5):1085-1087.

11. Goldman M, Compton C, Mittleman BB. Public-private partnerships as driving forces in the quest for innovative medicines. Clin Transl Med. 2013;2(1):2.

12. Trifirò G, Fourrier-Réglat A, Sturkenboom MC, et al. The EU-ADR project: preliminary results and perspective. Pharmacoepidemiol Drug Saf. 2009;18(12):1176–1184.8.

13. ENCePP Steering Group. ENCePP Guide on Methodological Standards in Pharmacoepidemiology (Revision 11). London: European Medicines Agency; 2023.

14. Cave A, Kurz X, Arlett P. Real-world data for regulatory decision making: challenges and possible solutions for Europe. Clin Pharmacol Ther. 2019;106(1):36–39.

15. European Medicines Agency. Guideline on Good Pharmacovigilance Practices (GVP) Module VIII - Post-authorisation safety studies. EMA/813938/2011 Rev. 3, 2017.

16. European Medicines Agency, Heads of Medicines Agencies. HMA-EMA Joint Big Data Task Force Phase II report: Evolving Data-Driven Regulation. Amsterdam: EMA; 2020 Jan.

17. European Medicines Agency, Committee for Medicinal Products for Human Use. Reflection paper on use of real-world data in non-interventional studies to generate real-world evidence for regulatory purposes. EMA/CHMP/150527/2024. Amsterdam: EMA; 2025 Mar.

18. Bussel J, Arnold DM, Grossbard E, et al. Fostamatinib for the treatment of adult persistent and chronic immune thrombocytopenia: results of two phase 3, randomized, placebo-controlled trials. Am J Hematol. 2018;93(7):921–930.

19. Williamson EJ, Walker AJ, Bhaskaran K, Bacon S, Bates C, Morton CE, et al. Factors associated with COVID-19-related death using OpenSAFELY. Nature. 2020;584(7821):430–436.

20. Woodcock A, Vestbo J, Bakerly ND, New J, Gibson JM, McCorkindale S, et al. Effectiveness of fluticasone furoate plus vilanterol on asthma control in clinical practice: an open-label, parallel group, randomised controlled trial. Lancet. 2017;390(10109):2247–2255.

21. Bakerly ND, Woodcock A, New JP, Gibson JM, Wu W, Leather D. The Salford Lung Study protocol: a pragmatic, randomised phase III real-world effectiveness trial in asthma. BMC Pulm Med. 2015;15:160.

22. Nishioka K, Makimura T, Ishiguro A, Nonaka T, Yamaguchi M, Uyama Y. Evolving acceptance and use of RWE for regulatory decision making on the benefit/risk assessment of a drug in Japan. Clin Pharmacol Ther. 2022;111(1):35–43.

23. Therapeutic Goods Administration. Real world evidence (RWE) and patient reported outcomes (PROs). Canberra: TGA; 2021.

24. Graves SE, Davidson D, Ingerson L, Ryan P, Griffith EC, McDermott BFJ, McElroy HJ, Pratt NL. The Australian Orthopaedic Association National Joint Replacement Registry. Med J Aust. 2004;180(5 Suppl):S31–S34.

25. Sankar C, Evans S, Meyer J, et al. Signal monitoring for adverse events following immunisation with COVID-19 vaccines during the SARS-CoV-2 pandemic: an evaluation of the South African surveillance system. Drug Saf. 2025;48(5):511–525.

26. Rajinikanth RG, Samanta S. The implications of waiving local clinical trials for drugs in India: a double-edged sword? Lancet Reg Health Southeast Asia. 2024;29:100490.

27. ICH. E9(R1) Addendum on Estimands and Sensitivity Analysis. 2019.

28. ICH. ICH M14 Guideline: General Principles on Planning, Designing, Analysing and Reporting of Non-interventional Studies that Utilise Real-World Data for Safety Assessment of Medicines. Step 4. 2025 Sep 4.

29. ICH. ICH reflection paper on pursuing opportunities for harmonisation in using real-world data to generate real-world evidence, with a focus on effectiveness of medicines. Geneva: ICH; 2024 Jun 4

# Chapter 11. RWE in Health Technology Assessment

Health Technology Assessment (HTA) represents a critical junction where clinical evidence meets economic and societal decision-making. While regulatory bodies focus primarily on safety and efficacy, HTA agencies evaluate whether a health technology provides sufficient value to justify its cost within a specific healthcare system. Real-world evidence has emerged as an increasingly important component of HTA submissions, complementing randomized controlled trial data with information about how technologies perform in routine clinical practice. This chapter explores the role of RWE in HTA processes, examining how different agencies worldwide incorporate real-world data into their assessments, the methodological considerations specific to HTA contexts, and practical guidance for generating and submitting RWE that meets HTA standards.

# 11.1. Understanding Health Technology Assessment

Health Technology Assessment is a multidisciplinary process that systematically evaluates the properties, effects, and impacts of health technologies. The primary purpose of HTA is to inform decision-making about the allocation of healthcare resources, including reimbursement decisions, pricing negotiations, and clinical guideline development. Unlike regulatory approval, which asks whether a technology is **safe and effective**, HTA asks whether it provides **good value for money** compared to existing alternatives.

HTA bodies operate at national and regional levels worldwide, each with their own methodologies, evidence requirements, and decision frameworks. The International Network of Agencies for Health Technology Assessment (INAHTA) coordinates more than 55 member organizations globally, while Health Technology Assessment International (HTAi) facilitates knowledge exchange among HTA professionals [1,2].

Despite this coordination, significant variation exists in how different agencies evaluate evidence and make recommendations. Table 11.1 provides a list of major HTA bodies.

The HTA process typically involves several key domains of evaluation. Clinical effectiveness assesses how well the technology works in practice compared to alternatives. Economic evaluation examines cost-effectiveness, cost-utility, or budget impact. Ethical considerations explore implications for patient autonomy, equity, and access. Organizational aspects consider how the technology fits within existing healthcare infrastructure. These domains collectively inform recommendations about whether and under what conditions a technology should be funded or adopted.

## 11.1.1. The Evolution of RWE in HTA

The incorporation of real-world evidence into HTA processes has evolved significantly over the past two decades. Historically, HTA agencies relied almost exclusively on randomized controlled trial data for clinical effectiveness inputs into economic models. This preference stemmed from concerns about bias, confounding, and data quality in observational studies.

**Table 11.1. Major HTA Agencies and Their RWE Requirements**

| Agency | Region/ Country | Primary Focus | RWE Acceptance Level | Key Guidelines |
|---|---|---|---|---|
| **NICE** | United Kingdom | Cost-effectiveness | High | NICE RWE Framework |
| **IQWiG** | Germany | Benefit assessment | Moderate | AMNOG Guidelines; IQWiG General Methods |
| **HAS** | France | Clinical benefit | Moderate | HAS Transparency Commission; HAS RWE Methodological Guide |
| **CDA-AMC (ex. CADTH)** | Canada | Comparative effectiveness | High | Guidance for Reporting Real-World Evidence (with Health Canada & INESSS) |
| **PBAC** | Australia | Cost-effectiveness | High | PBAC Guidelines |
| **AHRQ** | United States | Evidence synthesis | High | AHRQ EPC Methods; PCORI Methodology Standards |

However, several factors have driven increased acceptance of RWE in HTA contexts.

First, the limitations of RCT data for HTA purposes have become increasingly apparent. Randomized trials often exclude patients with comorbidities, elderly populations, or those on multiple medications - precisely the patients who will use the technology in routine practice. Trial settings may not reflect real-world clinical pathways, and follow-up periods are often too short to capture long-term outcomes relevant for economic evaluation. These limitations create evidence gaps that RWE can potentially address.

Second, the methodological quality of observational research has improved substantially in the last decade. Advanced statistical techniques for confounding control, including propensity score matching, instrumental variable analysis, and target trial emulation, have enhanced the credibility of RWE findings. Data quality has also improved with the digitization of health records and the development of large, linked databases suitable for research purposes.

Third, regulatory precedents have influenced HTA agencies. As regulators like the FDA and EMA have developed frameworks for accepting RWE in regulatory decision-making, HTA bodies have followed suit with their own guidance documents. Regulation (EU) 2021/2282 on Health Technology Assessment entered into force on 11 January 2022 and became applicable from 12 January 2025, explicitly acknowledging the role of real-world data in joint clinical assessments (EU JCA) [3].

The timeline of RWE acceptance in HTA reflects this evolution. In the early 2000s, RWE was rarely accepted for primary effectiveness claims. By 2010, agencies began accepting RWE for safety data and subgroup analyses. The period from 2015 to 2020 saw the development of formal RWE frameworks by major HTA agencies. Currently, RWE is routinely considered for multiple purposes including effectiveness extrapolation, comparator data, long-term outcomes, and subgroup analyses, though acceptance varies by agency and indication.

## 11.2. HTA Agency Frameworks for RWE

Different HTA agencies have developed distinct frameworks for evaluating and incorporating real-world evidence. Understanding these frameworks is essential for manufacturers preparing HTA submissions and researchers designing RWE studies intended to inform HTA decisions.

### 11.2.1. National Institute for Health and Care Excellence (NICE)

The United Kingdom's NICE has been among the most progressive HTA agencies in developing RWE guidance. The NICE Real-World Evidence Framework was first published in 2022 and represents a living document that has been updated multiple times since, including additions on external validity and transportability, qualitative research, and unstructured data [4]. NICE distinguishes between different types of RWE based on fitness for purpose, evaluating data quality, study design, and analytical methods.

NICE accepts RWE for several purposes in HTA submissions. These include supplementing clinical trial data when trials have limitations, providing evidence on long-term outcomes beyond trial follow-up, informing treatment patterns and resource use for economic modeling, and supporting evidence generation for managed access agreements. The agency has established a Real-World Evidence Advisory Service to provide pre-submission advice on RWE study plans.

A notable example of NICE's RWE acceptance is the technology appraisal TA766 (2022): the committee accepted Cancer Drugs Fund real-world data on subsequent treatment patterns following adjuvant pembrolizumab for resected stage 3 melanoma, using it on top of immature trial data from KEYNOTE-054, which the committee judged did not reflect NHS clinical practice. RWE from several sources were explicitly used to inform economic modelling of survival projections, post-progression therapy costs and outcomes, contributing to the positive recommendation [5].

### 11.2.2. Institute for Quality and Efficiency in Health Care (IQWiG)

Germany's IQWiG operates under the AMNOG (Act on the Reform of the Market for Medicinal Products) framework, which requires manufacturers to submit dossier assessments demonstrating added benefit compared to appropriate comparators [6]. IQWiG has traditionally maintained high standards for evidence quality, preferring randomized controlled trials for benefit assessments. However, the agency has increasingly accepted RWE when RCT data are unavailable or insufficient.

IQWiG's approach to RWE is characterized by rigorous assessment of study quality and risk of bias. The agency employs structured tools for evaluating observational studies and requires detailed documentation of data sources, patient selection, confounding control, and sensitivity analyses. RWE is particularly relevant in Germany for rare diseases where RCTs may be impractical, for comparator arms when active comparators are not included in trials, and for long-term safety and effectiveness data.

The German system presents unique challenges for RWE generation. The requirement to demonstrate added benefit versus a specific comparator defined by the Federal Joint Committee (G-BA) means that RWE studies must be carefully designed to match the appropriate comparator population. Additionally, IQWiG's preference for patient-relevant outcomes rather than surrogate endpoints requires RWE studies to capture meaningful clinical endpoints. Notably, both IQWiG and G-BA are active in shaping the EU JCA methodology through their participation in the Coordination Group.

### 11.2.3. Haute Autorité de Santé (HAS)

France's HAS operates through its Transparency Commission, which evaluates the clinical benefit and improvement in clinical benefit of health technologies. HAS developed guidance on the use of real-world studies for medicine and medical device evaluation, emphasizing the importance of study transparency and methodological rigor [7]. The agency accepts RWE for post-authorization studies, comparative effectiveness research, and evidence generation for re-evaluation of previously assessed technologies.

HAS places particular emphasis on the French national health data system (SNDS), which links claims data, hospital discharge data, and cause of death information for virtually the entire French population. This resource enables large-scale observational studies with long follow-up periods. HAS has accepted RWE from SNDS for multiple technology assessments, particularly in oncology and rare diseases where patient populations are small and trial data are limited.

### 11.2.4. Canada's Drug Agency / CDA-AMC (formerly CADTH)

In 2023 the Canadian Drug Agency (CDA-AMC) published its Guidance for Reporting Real-World Evidence, developed in partnership with Health Canada and the Institut national d'excellence en santé et en services sociaux *(INESSS)* [8]. This guidance outlines principles for generating, analyzing, and interpreting RWE for HTA and regulatory decision-making purposes, emphasizing fitness for purpose, transparency, and reproducibility.

CDA-AMC accepts RWE for multiple purposes including informing clinical input parameters for economic models, providing evidence on treatment patterns and resource use, supporting extrapolation of trial outcomes, and informing subgroup analyses. The Canadian context presents specific considerations for RWE generation, including provincial variation in healthcare delivery and data availability. CDA-AMC encourages the use of multiple data sources when possible and emphasizes validating findings across different datasets.

### 11.2.5. Pharmaceutical Benefits Advisory Committee (PBAC)

Australia's PBAC evaluates medicines for inclusion on the Pharmaceutical Benefits Scheme based on comparative effectiveness and cost-effectiveness [9]. The PBAC Guidelines allow non-randomized evidence and provide methodological expectations (e.g., transparency, stepped approach, indirect comparisons). RWE is particularly important in the Australian context for comparing new technologies with existing treatments that may not have been directly compared in randomized trials.

PBAC has accepted RWE for several purposes including providing evidence on relative effectiveness when head-to-head trials are unavailable, informing long-term outcomes beyond trial follow-up, supporting evidence for rare diseases where RCTs are challenging, and validating trial findings in Australian populations. The agency emphasizes the importance of addressing potential biases and conducting sensitivity analyses to assess the robustness of RWE findings.

## 11.3. EU Joint Clinical Assessment

Regulation (EU) 2021/2282 on Health Technology Assessment entered into force in 2022 and became applicable across all 27 EU Member States 2025. Its centerpiece is the Joint Clinical Assessment (JCA): a centralized, EU-level evaluation of the relative clinical effectiveness of health technologies conducted in parallel with the EMA marketing authorization review [3]. The JCA is being introduced in phases: new oncology medicines and advanced therapy medicinal products (ATMPs) i.e. cell & gene therapies and tissue-engineered products from 2025, orphan medicines from 2028, and all new centrally authorized products from 2030. Critically, the JCA is limited to clinical assessment only - pricing, reimbursement, and economic evaluation remain the sovereign competence of individual Member States, which must give "due consideration" to JCA reports in their national processes but are not bound by its conclusions.

Although RCTs remain the primary evidence source for JCA, RWE plays several important supporting roles. For oncology and ATMPs - the initial JCA scope - overall survival data are frequently immature at the time of marketing authorization; RWE from cancer registries and linked databases can supplement trial data with extended follow-up. RWE is also used to characterize real-world patient populations across diverse European healthcare systems, to provide comparative effectiveness data against country-specific standard-of-care comparators not studied in pivotal trials, and to support natural history documentation in rare disease assessments.

A distinct operational challenge for the JCA is timing: because the dossier is submitted shortly after EMA authorization, any RWE intended for the JCA must be planned and largely completed during clinical development, not post-launch. The compressed submission window - approximately 90 - 100 days after PICO confirmation - leaves no time to commission new studies. Early integrated evidence planning and, where available, engagement through Joint Scientific Consultations before trial lock are therefore essential for manufacturers targeting major European markets.

The JCA does not remove the need for country-specific RWE. National HTA bodies continue to conduct their own economic and relative-effectiveness evaluations using the JCA report as one input, and managed access arrangements in individual Member States will continue to generate post-launch RWE as they do today. The JCA thus functions as a new upstream layer in the evidence generation pathway rather than a replacement for existing national processes, reinforcing the importance of multi-country, comparator-rich RWE strategies that can serve both the JCA dossier and subsequent national submissions.

## 11.4. Methodological Considerations for HTA-Focused RWE

Generating RWE for HTA purposes requires careful attention to methodological considerations that may differ from those relevant for regulatory submissions. HTA agencies focus on comparative effectiveness and economic evaluation, which creates specific requirements for RWE study design and analysis. Table 11.2 provides a summary of key methodological requirements of HTA bodies for RWE studies.

### 11.4.1. Comparator Selection and Validity

One of the most critical considerations for HTA-focused RWE is the selection of appropriate comparators. Unlike regulatory submissions where placebo-controlled trials may be acceptable, HTA requires comparison with relevant alternatives used in routine practice. This creates challenges when the technology of interest has not been directly compared with all relevant comparators in randomized trials.

RWE studies can address this gap by providing comparative effectiveness data against multiple active comparators. However, this requires careful attention to confounding control, as patients receiving different treatments in routine practice may differ systematically in ways that affect outcomes. Propensity score methods, including matching, weighting, and stratification, are commonly employed to address observed confounding. Unmeasured confounding remains a concern and should be addressed through sensitivity analyses and discussion of limitations.

The target trial emulation framework has gained traction for HTA-focused RWE studies. This approach involves explicitly designing observational studies to emulate the protocol of a hypothetical randomized trial, including clear eligibility criteria, treatment assignment rules, follow-up periods, and outcome definitions [10]. This framework enhances transparency and helps HTA reviewers assess the validity of RWE findings.

**Table 11.2. Key Methodological Requirements for HTA RWE Studies**

| Domain | Key Requirements |
|---|---|
| **Study Design** | Target trial emulation; clear eligibility criteria; predefined analysis plan; protocol registration prior to analysis |
| **Comparator Selection** | Relevant to HTA jurisdiction; appropriate confounding control; multiple sensitivity analyses; reflects current standard of care |
| **Outcomes** | Patient-relevant endpoints (e.g., overall survival, QoL, function); sufficient follow-up; validated measures aligned with HTA agency preferences |
| **Data Quality** | Source documentation; validation procedures; completeness assessment; description of known limitations |
| **Transparency** | Protocol registration; pre-specified statistical analysis plan; full results including sensitivity analyses; clear limitation disclosure; code availability where possible |

## 11.4.2. Outcome Selection and Measurement

HTA agencies prioritize patient-relevant outcomes over surrogate endpoints. While regulatory submissions may accept surrogate markers like progression-free survival or biomarker responses, HTA bodies typically require evidence on overall survival, quality of life, functional status, or other outcomes that matter to patients and healthcare systems.

RWE studies for HTA must therefore capture appropriate endpoints that align with HTA agency requirements. This may require linkage of multiple data sources to obtain comprehensive outcome information. For example, cancer registry data may provide survival information, while claims data capture healthcare utilization, and patient-reported outcome measures assess quality of life. The feasibility of capturing these outcomes varies by data source and healthcare system.

### 11.4.3. Generalizability and Representativeness

HTA agencies evaluate technologies for specific populations within their healthcare systems. RWE studies should therefore demonstrate that the study population is representative of the population for whom the technology will be used. This includes consideration of demographic characteristics, disease severity, comorbidities, and prior treatments.

Subgroup analyses are often requested by HTA agencies to inform decisions about specific patient populations. RWE studies can provide evidence for subgroups that were underrepresented in clinical trials, such as elderly patients, those with comorbidities, or specific genetic subtypes. However, subgroup analyses in observational studies require careful interpretation due to reduced sample sizes and potential for residual confounding.

### 11.4.4. Data Quality and Transparency

HTA agencies place strong emphasis on data quality and study transparency. RWE submissions should include detailed documentation of data sources, including data collection methods, coverage, completeness, and known limitations. Data validation procedures should be described, including any checks for data accuracy and consistency.

Protocol registration and pre-specification of analyses enhance credibility of RWE findings. Several HTA agencies encourage or require registration of observational studies in public registries before analysis begins. This reduces concerns about selective reporting and data-driven analyses.

## 11.4.5. External Control Arms and Synthetic Comparators

An increasingly important methodological approach in HTA-relevant RWE is the use of external control arms (ECAs), also referred to as synthetic control arms or historical control arms. ECAs use patient-level data from external sources - including disease registries, natural history studies, or prior clinical trials - to construct a comparator group in settings where a concurrent randomized control arm is impractical or ethically infeasible. This approach is particularly relevant for rare diseases, pediatric indications, and ATMPs where the patient population is small or where randomization to placebo would be unethical.

The construction of credible ECAs requires rigorous attention to several methodological principles. External control patients must be drawn from a population comparable to the treatment group in terms of eligibility criteria, baseline characteristics, follow-up timing, and outcome measurement. Propensity score weighting and matching methods are commonly applied to minimize baseline imbalances, and sensitivity analyses addressing unmeasured confounding are essential.

The NICE and CDA-AMC have accepted ECA evidence in submissions for orphan and rare disease indications when no alternative comparator design was feasible. The case of onasemnogene abeparvovec (see 11.9.2), where natural history cohort data served as the primary basis for contextualizing single-arm trial results in the CADTH review, illustrates both the value and the limitations of this approach: while ECAs can provide essential comparative context, the resulting cost-effectiveness estimates carry substantial uncertainty that must be explicitly characterized in economic models. As JCA submissions are required to include relevant comparator data for all EU member states - many of which may have distinct standard-of-care comparators - the ECA methodology will become an increasingly prominent component of integrated evidence strategies for rare disease technologies.

## 11.5. RWE in Economic Evaluation

Economic evaluation is a core component of HTA, and RWE plays multiple roles in informing economic models. Understanding how RWE contributes to economic evaluation is essential for designing studies that meet HTA requirements.

### 11.5.1. Clinical Input Parameters

Economic models require estimates of clinical parameters including treatment effectiveness, survival, adverse event rates, and treatment discontinuation. While randomized trial data often provide the primary source for these parameters, RWE can supplement or replace trial data in several circumstances.

When trial follow-up is insufficient to characterize long-term outcomes, RWE can provide extended follow-up data for survival extrapolation. This is particularly relevant in oncology, where overall survival may extend years beyond trial follow-up periods. RWE from cancer registries or linked databases can inform the tail of survival curves used in economic models.

Treatment patterns and sequencing information from RWE informs modeling of subsequent therapies and their costs and outcomes. In many disease areas, patients receive multiple lines of therapy, and the effectiveness and cost of subsequent treatments affect the overall cost-effectiveness of the initial therapy. Claims data and electronic health records can provide detailed information on treatment pathways.

### 11.5.2. Resource Use and Costs

RWE is particularly valuable for estimating resource use and costs, which are rarely captured comprehensively in clinical trials. Healthcare utilization patterns vary across settings and countries, and trial protocols may not reflect routine practice in terms of monitoring frequency, supportive care, or management of adverse events.

Claims databases provide detailed information on healthcare utilization including hospitalizations, outpatient visits, procedures, and medications. When linked with clinical data, these sources can provide comprehensive cost information for economic models. However, cost data must be carefully validated and may require adjustment to reflect the specific HTA jurisdiction's pricing and reimbursement structures.

### 11.5.3. Model Validation and Calibration

RWE can be used to validate and calibrate economic models, increasing confidence in model predictions. External validation involves comparing model outputs with observed outcomes from RWE sources not used in model development. This assesses whether the model accurately predicts real-world outcomes. HTA agencies increasingly expect some form of model validation using RWE.

## 11.6. Managed Access and Evidence Development

Many HTA agencies have developed mechanisms for conditional reimbursement while additional evidence is generated. These managed access agreements create opportunities for systematic RWE generation that directly informs HTA decisions. Figure 11.1 shows a typical managed access evidence generation cycle.

### 11.6.1. NICE Managed Access Agreements

NICE's managed access pathway allows technologies to be recommended for use while additional evidence is collected to address uncertainties. This approach is particularly relevant for technologies with promising but uncertain evidence, such as those approved based on surrogate endpoints or small patient populations. RWE collection under managed access agreements must be systematic and designed to address specific evidence gaps identified during the HTA review [11].

Several oncology therapies have been appraised through NICE's managed access pathway, with RWE collected through cancer registries and hospital data systems. The evidence generated has informed subsequent reassessments, with some technologies receiving full recommendations and others being withdrawn from the pathway when evidence failed to demonstrate sufficient value [12].

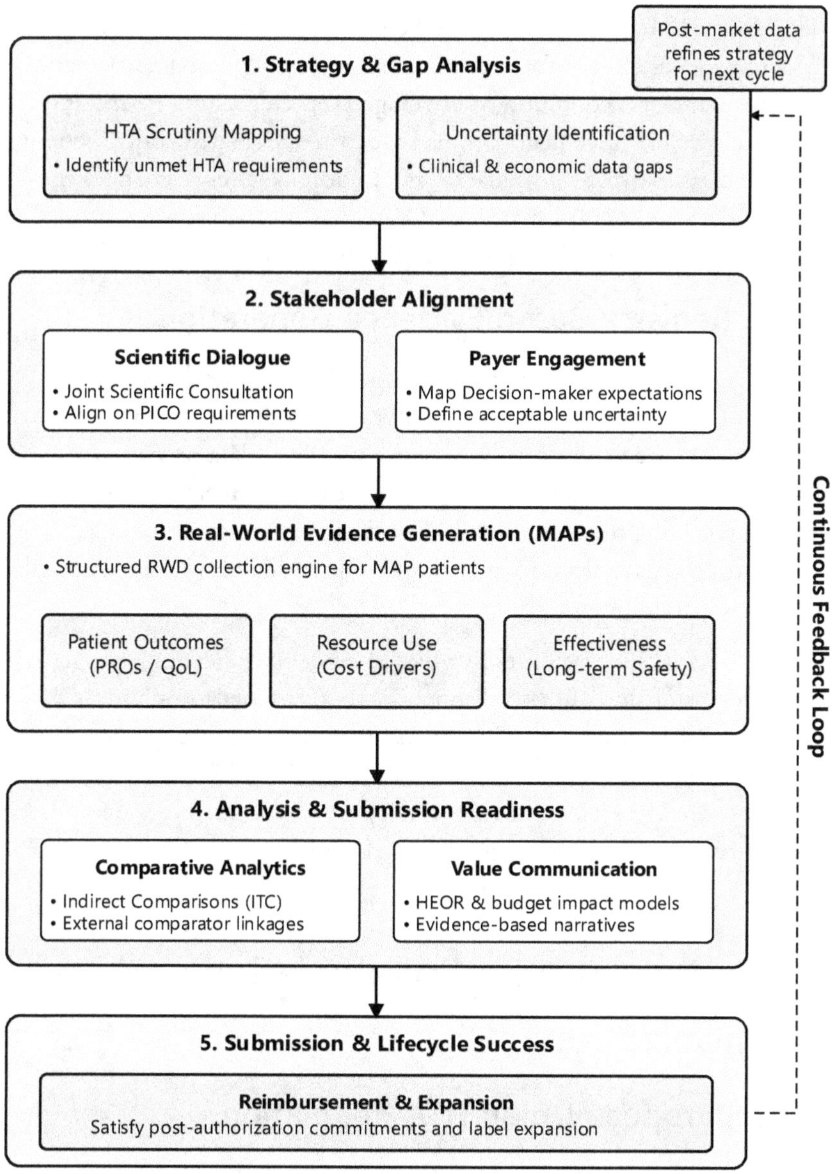


**Figure 11.1. Managed Access Evidence Generation Cycle**

### 11.6.2. Coverage with Evidence Development

Similar mechanisms exist in other jurisdictions. The Centers for Medicare and Medicaid Services in the United States offers Coverage with Evidence Development for certain technologies, requiring participation in data collection as a condition of coverage [13]. Germany's AMNOG system allows for price negotiations based on anticipated added benefit, with the possibility of re-evaluation if additional evidence changes the benefit assessment [14]. Australia's PBAC has mechanisms for listing medicines with restrictions while additional evidence is collected.

### 11.6.3. Registry-Based Evidence Generation

Disease-specific and product-specific registries represent important infrastructure for RWE generation under managed access arrangements. Registries can systematically collect data on patient characteristics, treatment patterns, outcomes, and adverse events for patients receiving the technology. Well-designed registries include standardized data collection instruments, clear eligibility criteria, and plans for long-term follow-up.

Several successful registry-based evidence generation programs exist internationally. The Swedish national quality registries have generated RWE informing HTA decisions for multiple technologies. The United Kingdom's Cancer Drugs Fund has collected RWE on oncology therapies through systematic data collection. These examples demonstrate the feasibility and value of registry-based evidence generation for HTA purposes.

## 11.7. International Collaboration and Harmonization

### 11.7.1. European Union HTA Regulation

The European Union's Regulation (EU) 2021/2282 on Health Technology Assessment represents a significant development in HTA harmonization across Europe [3]. The regulation establishes a framework for joint clinical assessments of new medicines and medical devices through the Member State Coordination Group on Health Technology Assessment (HTACG), reducing duplication of effort across member states.

The JCA framework supports the role of real-world data in assessments. Member States are expected to collaborate on RWE generation and sharing, potentially creating larger datasets for analysis. However, the regulation maintains national sovereignty over pricing and reimbursement decisions, meaning full economic evaluation requirements will continue to vary across countries, and national HTA bodies will still conduct their own assessments using JCA reports as one input alongside country-specific evidence.

### 11.7.2. International HTA Networks

Organizations like INAHTA and HTAi facilitate international collaboration on HTA methods and evidence standards. The International Society for Pharmacoeconomics and Outcomes Research (ISPOR) has developed good practices for RWE that are widely referenced by HTA agencies. Adoption of common standards enhances the acceptability of RWE across jurisdictions.

Parallel scientific advice processes allow manufacturers to seek guidance from multiple HTA agencies simultaneously. The EMA and several HTA agencies offer parallel advice procedures where manufacturers can receive coordinated feedback on evidence generation plans, including RWE studies.

### 11.7.3. Challenges in International RWE Harmonization

Despite collaboration efforts, significant challenges remain. Data privacy regulations vary across jurisdictions, with the EU's General Data Protection Regulation (GDPR) creating specific requirements for data processing and transfer that complicate international data pooling. Healthcare system differences affect both data availability and the generalizability of RWE findings. Initiatives like the Observational Health Data Sciences and Informatics (OHDSI) community are working to standardize observational data, but adoption remains incomplete.

# 11.8. Practical Guidance for RWE in HTA Submissions

## 11.8.1. Pre-Submission Planning

Early engagement with HTA agencies is strongly recommended for RWE intended to support HTA submissions. Many agencies offer pre-submission advice services where manufacturers can discuss evidence plans and receive feedback on acceptability. When planning RWE studies for HTA, consider the specific questions the HTA agency is likely to ask: What comparators are relevant in this jurisdiction? What outcomes are prioritized? What uncertainties exist in the current evidence base? Table 11.3 provides an RWE submission checklist for HTA.

## 11.8.2. Study Design Considerations

For HTA-focused RWE studies, target trial emulation provides a useful framework for design - whenever relevant. Explicitly specify the eligibility criteria, treatment assignment rules, follow-up period, and outcomes to be measured. Comparator selection requires careful attention to the HTA context: identify the appropriate comparator based on current clinical practice in the target jurisdiction. Sample size calculations should account for the need to detect clinically meaningful differences.

## 11.8.3. Analysis and Reporting

Statistical analysis plans should be comprehensive and pre-specified. Include detailed descriptions of methods for confounding control, handling of missing data, subgroup analyses, and sensitivity analyses. Address potential biases explicitly in the analysis and reporting. Reporting should follow established guidelines such as the RECORD statement for studies using routinely collected health data [15].

## 11.8.4. Submission Documentation

HTA submissions should include comprehensive documentation of RWE studies: the study protocol, statistical analysis plan, data dictionary, analysis code (where possible), and full results including sensitivity analyses. Some agencies now expect analysis code to be made available for independent verification. Economic model documentation should clearly indicate which parameters are informed by RWE and provide sensitivity analyses showing the impact of RWE uncertainty on cost-effectiveness results.

**Table 11.3. RWE Submission Checklist for HTA**

| Component | Required Elements | Common Pitfalls |
|---|---|---|
| **Study Protocol** | Objectives, design, eligibility criteria, outcomes, pre-registration | Vague objectives; post-hoc design changes; no registration |
| **Data Source Description** | Coverage, completeness, validation procedures, access permissions | Insufficient detail on limitations; no validation documentation |
| **Analysis Plan** | Confounding control methods, sensitivity analyses, missing data strategy | Inadequate bias assessment; no sensitivity analyses |
| **Results Reporting** | Full results including subgroup analyses; adherence to RECORD or similar | Selective reporting; insufficient detail on negative or null findings |
| **Economic Model Integration** | Parameter sources clearly identified; uncertainty ranges; model validation | Unclear contribution of RWE; no sensitivity analysis for RWE inputs |

# 11.9. Case Examples

## 11.9.1. Nivolumab for Adjuvant Melanoma - NICE Technology Appraisal

Nivolumab, a PD-1 checkpoint inhibitor, was submitted to NICE for adjuvant treatment of completely resected melanoma with lymph node involvement or metastatic disease. The pivotal evidence came from CheckMate 238, a randomized phase 3 trial comparing nivolumab with ipilimumab that demonstrated significantly improved recurrence-free survival [15]. However, overall survival data were immature at the time of submission, and no direct randomized comparison with routine surveillance - the then standard of care in the NHS - was available. NICE issued TA558 in 2019, recommending nivolumab within the Cancer

Drugs Fund under a managed access agreement precisely because of this overall survival uncertainty [16]. Data collection requirements specified continued long-term follow-up of patients receiving nivolumab, including those who subsequently developed advanced disease and received further treatment.

RWE played a dual role in this case.

- **Cancer Drugs Fund** data collected during the managed access period contributed to the evidence base reviewed at reassessment.
- **Indirect treatment comparison** methods, drawing on observational data for the ipilimumab arm as a common comparator, were used to bridge the gap between the available trial data and the NHS-relevant comparator.

At reassessment (TA684, 2021), NICE moved nivolumab to routine commissioning, concluding that the most plausible cost-effectiveness estimates fell within acceptable thresholds once additional survival data had been incorporated. This case illustrates how managed access enables conditional approval where RCT follow-up is insufficient, with systematically collected RWE directly informing the decision to convert to full recommendation.

### 11.9.2. Onasemnogene Abeparvovec for Spinal Muscular Atrophy - CADTH/CDA-AMC Review

Onasemnogene abeparvovec, an adeno-associated virus-based gene replacement therapy for 5q spinal muscular atrophy (SMA), was reviewed by CADTH in 2021 with one of the most limited evidence bases encountered in a major HTA submission [17]. The pivotal study, STR1VE-US, was a single-arm phase 3 trial enrolling just 22 patients with SMA type 1. No head-to-head randomized comparison with nusinersen - the main active comparator - was feasible, and the CADTH review acknowledged that an anchored indirect treatment comparison was not possible given the small sample size and absence of a common comparator arm.

RWE contributed in two critical ways:

- Natural history cohort data provided the external comparator against which the single-arm trial results were interpreted, enabling a contextualization of the profound motor milestone improvements observed;
- Early access program data, alongside the RESTORE registry launched in 2018, began generating longer-term effectiveness and safety evidence to address the substantial extrapolation uncertainty in the economic model [18].

CADTH concluded that the cost-effectiveness of onasemnogene abeparvovec was highly uncertain, with an estimated incremental cost-effectiveness ratio exceeding $334,000 per QALY compared with best supportive care at the submitted price, driven almost entirely by extrapolation beyond observed trial data [19]. Despite this, the therapy received a conditional recommendation in several Canadian provinces subject to managed entry arrangements requiring price reduction and continued real-world data collection. This case demonstrates the value of natural history RWE and registry infrastructure in rare disease HTA, where randomized controlled trials are inherently limited in size and design, and where RWE is often the only available basis for contextualizing single-arm trial results.

### 11.9.3. Infliximab Biosimilar CT-P13 - Indication Extrapolation Supported by RWE

CT-P13, the first biosimilar monoclonal antibody to be approved by the EMA (2013) and subsequently by the FDA (2016), provides a landmark example of RWE supporting indication extrapolation in HTA [20]. The marketing authorization was based on two pivotal phase 3 trials - PLANETRA in rheumatoid arthritis and PLANETAS in ankylosing spondylitis - neither of which enrolled patients with inflammatory bowel disease (IBD), psoriatic arthritis, or plaque psoriasis. Approval for all six indications of the originator infliximab was granted on the basis of extrapolation. This extrapolation generated substantial clinical hesitancy, particularly among gastroenterologists concerned about the adequacy of RA as a sensitive clinical model for IBD indications where infliximab has distinct mechanisms of action.

RWE played a decisive role in validating indication extrapolation across subsequent HTA and reimbursement decisions. A large nationwide cohort study in patients with ulcerative colitis treated with CT-P13 versus originator infliximab - using routinely collected registry and claims data - demonstrated equivalent effectiveness with a hazard ratio of 1.04(95% CI, 0.90-1.20) within pre-specified equivalence margins [21]. The multinational NOR-SWITCH study, a prospective randomized double-blind non-inferiority switch trial, further supported interchangeability across multiple indications [22]. Pooled observational analyses of long-term real-world outcomes across RA, IBD, and ankylosing spondylitis populations subsequently provided the evidence base that informed HTA decisions in multiple European countries, supporting broader formulary adoption and substitution policies. This case illustrates how RWE can progress from hypothesis-generating to decision-grade evidence over time, particularly for biosimilars where post-authorization data are essential to build clinician and payer confidence in extrapolated indications.

## 11.10. Conclusion

Real-world evidence has become an integral component of Health Technology Assessment, complementing randomized trial data with information about how technologies perform in routine clinical practice. Major HTA agencies worldwide have developed frameworks for evaluating and incorporating RWE, though acceptance levels and specific requirements vary across jurisdictions. NICE, CDA-AMC, and PBAC have been among the most progressive in developing comprehensive RWE guidance, whereas IQWiG and HAS maintain more selective approaches while increasingly accepting RWE for specific purposes.

The EU JCA, introduces a new upstream layer of centralized clinical assessment for oncology and ATMPs across all Member States. While the JCA does not replace national economic evaluations, it reshapes the evidence generation timeline: RWE intended for the JCA must be ready at the time of marketing authorization rather than developed post-launch, reinforcing the importance of integrating RWE planning into early clinical development.

Methodological rigor remains paramount. Studies should employ robust designs including (when relevant) target trial emulation, appropriate confounding control, and comprehensive sensitivity analyses. Transparency in protocol registration, analysis planning, and reporting enhances credibility. International collaboration on RWE standards continues to evolve.

For manufacturers, researchers, and HTA professionals, understanding the role of RWE in HTA is essential for navigating the evolving evidence landscape. Thoughtful generation and transparent reporting of RWE can enhance the evidence base for HTA decisions, ultimately supporting more informed allocation of healthcare resources and improved patient access to valuable technologies.

## References

1. INAHTA. International Network of Agencies for Health Technology Assessment. Available from: https://www.inahta.org

2. HTAi. Health Technology Assessment international. Available from: https://htai.org.

3. European Union. Regulation (EU) 2021/2282 of the European Parliament and of the Council of 15 December 2021 on health technology assessment and amending Directive 2011/24/EU. Official Journal of the European Union. 2021;L458:1–45.

4. National Institute for Health and Care Excellence. NICE real-world evidence framework. London: NICE; 2022

5. National Institute for Health and Care Excellence. Pembrolizumab for adjuvant treatment of completely resected stage 3 melanoma [TA766]. London: NICE; 2022.

6. Institute for Quality and Efficiency in Health Care. General methods for the assessment of the relation of benefits to harms, version 7.0. Cologne: IQWiG; 2022.

7. Haute Autorité de Santé. Real-world studies for the assessment of medicinal products and medical devices - Methodological guide. Saint-Denis La Plaine: HAS; June 2021.

8. Canada's Drug Agency (CDA-AMC; formerly CADTH); Health Canada; INESSS. Guidance for Reporting Real-World Evidence. Ottawa: CDA-AMC; May 2023.

9. Pharmaceutical Benefits Advisory Committee. Guidelines for preparing submissions to the PBAC (Version 5.0). Canberra: Australian Government Department of Health; 2022.

10. Hernán MA, Robins JM. Using big data to emulate a target trial when a randomized trial is not available. Am J Epidemiol. 2016;183(8):758–764.

11. National Institute for Health and Care Excellence. NICE health technology evaluations: the manual [PMG36]. London: NICE; 2022.

12. Aggarwal A, Fojo T, Chamberlain C, et al. Do patient access schemes for high-cost cancer drugs deliver value to society? lessons from the NHS Cancer Drugs Fund. Ann Oncol. 2017;28(8):1738–1750.

13. Centers for Medicare and Medicaid Services. Coverage with Evidence Development guidance document. Baltimore: CMS; 2024.

14. Gemeinsamer Bundesausschuss (Federal Joint Committee). Verfahrensordnung des Gemeinsamen Bundesausschusses, Kapitel 5: Bewertung des Nutzens von Arzneimitteln mit neuen Wirkstoffen gemäß § 35a SGB V [Rules of Procedure of the Federal Joint Committee, Chapter 5: Benefit Assessment of Medicinal Products with New Active Substances]. Berlin: G-BA; 2011.

15. Benchimol EI, Smeeth L, Guttmann A, et al. The REporting of studies Conducted using Observational Routinely-collected health Data (RECORD) statement. PLoS Medicine. 2015;12(10):e1001885.

15. Weber JS, Mandala M, Del Vecchio M, et al. Adjuvant nivolumab versus ipilimumab in resected stage III or IV melanoma. N Engl J Med. 2017;377(19):1824–1835.

16. National Institute for Health and Care Excellence. Nivolumab for adjuvant treatment of completely resected melanoma with lymph node involvement or metastatic disease. Technology Appraisal TA558. London: NICE; January 2019. [Managed access agreement]

17. Canadian Agency for Drugs and Technologies in Health. Clinical review report: onasemnogene abeparvovec (Zolgensma). Ottawa: CADTH; May 2021.

18. Servais L, Day JW, De Vivo DC, et al. Real-world outcomes in patients with spinal muscular atrophy treated with onasemnogene abeparvovec monotherapy: findings from the RESTORE registry. J Neuromuscul Dis. 2024;11(2):391–402.

19. Canadian Agency for Drugs and Technologies in Health. Pharmacoeconomic report: onasemnogene abeparvovec (Zolgensma). Ottawa: CADTH; May 2021.

20. European Medicines Agency. Assessment report: Remsima (infliximab). CHMP/589422/2013. London: EMA; 2013

21. Gower-Rousseau C, Dauchet L, Vernier-Massouille G, et al. Real-world comparative effectiveness of biosimilar CT-P13 versus reference infliximab in ulcerative colitis: a nationwide cohort study. Aliment Pharmacol Ther. 2019;50(6):651-660.

22. Jørgensen KK, Olsen IC, Goll GL, et al. Switching from originator infliximab to biosimilar CT-P13 compared with maintained treatment with originator infliximab (NOR-SWITCH): a 52-week, randomised, double-blind, non-inferiority trial. Lancet. 2017;389(10086):2304–2316.

# Chapter 12. RWE in Clinical and Operational Decision-Making

Real-world evidence (RWE) is no longer confined to regulatory submissions or academic inquiry - it is increasingly embedded in the day-to-day decisions that shape clinical care and health system operations. The shift from episodic evaluation to continuous, data-informed practice reflects broader evolutions in healthcare delivery: value-based payment models, integrated health systems, patient-centered care pathways, and the proliferation of digital health tools.

This chapter explores how clinicians, hospital administrators, regional health authorities, and integrated care teams harness RWE for three core purposes: frontline clinical decision support, operational optimization, and quality improvement initiatives.

We begin by examining the use of RWE within hospitals, especially in complex domains such as antimicrobial stewardship, oncology pathways, acute care risk stratification, and post-marketing drug safety. We then broaden the view to integrated care settings - where multiple providers across primary, secondary, and community care coordinate services - and show how RWE supports care continuity and population health management. Finally, we detail how quality improvement (QI) programs, from Lean and Six Sigma initiatives to national audit cycles, rely on RWE to set baselines, identify variation, and sustain gains. Throughout, we present concrete examples from the United States, the European Union, and other regions to illustrate the scalability and adaptability of RWE approaches.

## 12.1. Hospitals

Hospitals generate vast amounts of structured and unstructured real-world data (RWD) - electronic health records (EHRs), laboratory results, medication administration records, imaging archives, and billing codes. When these data are curated and analyzed with appropriate methodological rigor, they yield evidence that informs clinical protocols, resource allocation, and risk mitigation strategies.

### 12.1.1. Clinical Decision Support Embedded in Workflow

A growing number of institutions have moved from static clinical guidelines to dynamic, data-driven decision support tools. The Targeted Real-time Early Warning System (TREWS), developed at Johns Hopkins Hospital, was among the first large-scale deployments of a machine learning (ML)-based alert for septic shock. By integrating vital signs, laboratory trends, and nursing assessments, TREWScore - the underlying algorithm - identifies patients at risk of deterioration a median of 28 hours before onset [1]. In a subsequent prospective evaluation across five US hospital sites monitoring over 590,000 patients, provider interaction with the TREWS alert within three hours was associated with an 18.7% adjusted relative reduction in in-hospital mortality and significant reductions in organ failure and length of stay compared with patients whose alerts were not promptly confirmed [2]. An earlier single-center randomized clinical trial at University of California, San Franciso (UCSF) provided initial interventional support for ML-based sepsis surveillance, showing improvements in mortality and length of stay in a small ICU cohort [3]. Because models of this class derive their parameters from local patient trajectories rather than from trial populations, their performance adapts to the institution's case mix and documentation patterns - underscoring the advantage of locally generated RWE.

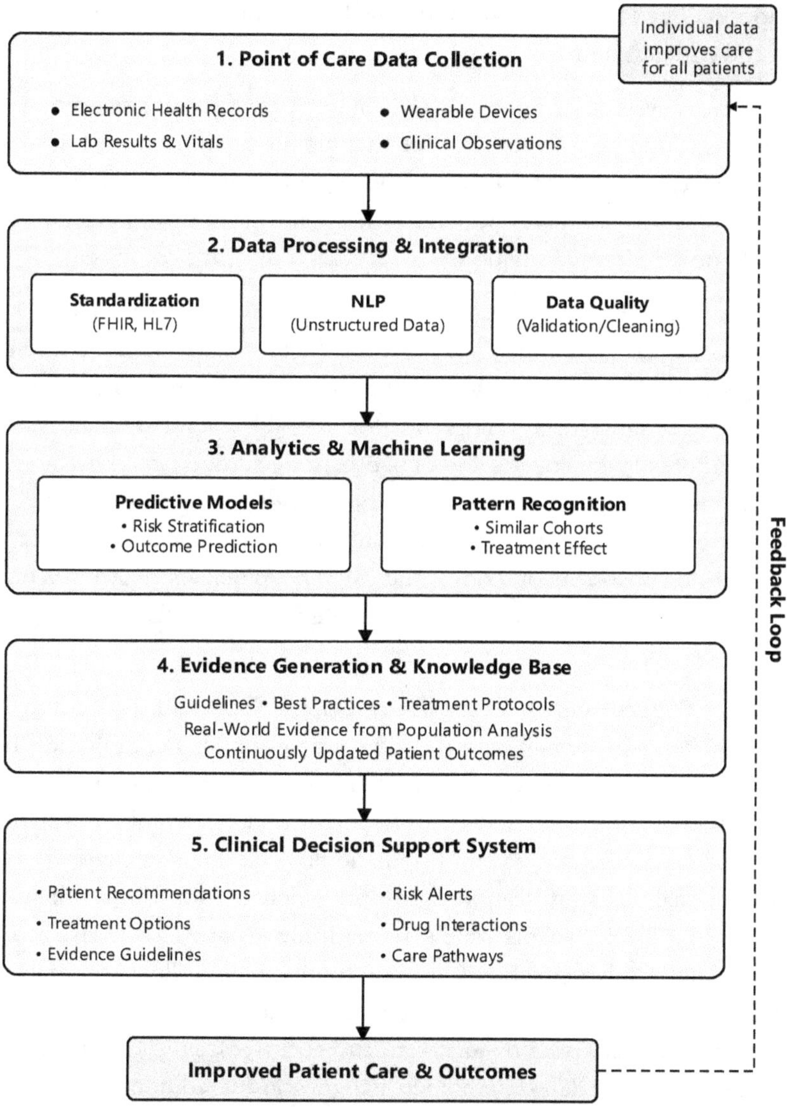


**Figure 12.1 Flow Diagram from Point of Care to Decision Support**

shows a flow diagram of data from point of care to decision support. The individual patient data will contribute to the improvement of the entire system.

A systematic review of clinical deterioration early warning systems found consistent evidence that higher-fidelity alert tools, when embedded directly into EHR workflows, improved the timeliness of clinical response. However, heterogeneity across study designs limited the final pooled effect estimation [4].

In Europe, the Dutch National Intensive Care Evaluation (NICE) registry combines ICU data from all participating Dutch ICUs into a national dashboard that compares observed versus expected mortality, length of stay, and ventilator days [5]. Each ICU receives quarterly feedback reports and benchmarking summaries, enabling rapid detection of outlier performance and prompting root cause reviews. Importantly, the registry is linked to hospital discharge data, allowing analyses of post-ICU outcomes such as rehospitalization and functional status at 90 days - an example of how longitudinal RWD supports outcome-oriented decision making.

A persistent challenge in deploying RWE-enabled decision support tools is the risk of embedding and amplifying existing health inequities. Models trained predominantly on data from well-resourced academic medical centers may underperform in community hospitals or for under-represented patient populations. A landmark analysis of a commercial risk stratification algorithm widely used in US health systems found that black patients were systematically assigned lower risk scores than equally ill white patients, leading to inequitable allocation of care management resources [6]. Prospective bias auditing, disaggregated performance reporting by race, sex, and socioeconomic status, and inclusive training datasets are increasingly considered non-negotiable prerequisites for any RWE-enabled clinical tool [7].

### 12.1.2. Antimicrobial Stewardship and Infection Prevention

Antimicrobial resistance (AMR) remains a global threat, and stewardship programs now rely heavily on RWE to guide empiric therapy. The US Centers for Disease Control and Prevention (CDC) launched the Antibiotic Resistance Laboratory Network (AR Lab Network), which links phenotypic resistance test results from nationwide public health laboratories to hospital EHRs, generating localized antibiograms that are refreshed quarterly [8].

In the United Kingdom, the Royal College of General Practitioners' TARGET (Treat Antibiotics Responsibly, Guide, Educate, Review and Trust) program uses linked primary care and hospital records to monitor prescribing trends and map resistance patterns regionally [9]. The program identified patterns of fluoroquinolone overuse in primary care clinics serving semi-rural populations, prompting targeted education and audit feedback interventions. National surveillance data from the English Surveillance Programme for Antimicrobial Utilisation and Resistance (ESPAUR) have documented progressive reductions in fluoroquinolone prescribing in primary care following such targeted programs, without evidence of compromised infection outcomes [10].

### 12.1.3. Oncology Pathways and Treatment Sequencing

In oncology, where therapeutic options proliferate, RWE helps define pragmatic treatment pathways. Flatiron Health's de-identified EHR database, covering over two million US cancer patients, has been used to characterize real-world utilization and outcomes of immune checkpoint inhibitors in non-small cell lung cancer (NSCLC). Analyses have revealed that patients treated in routine practice were older and had more often history of smoking as compared to those in pivotal clinical trials. They generally achieved survival outcomes broadly consistent with those reported in trials, while also demonstrating the substantially greater heterogeneity of the real-world population and the necessity of taking into consideration the subgroups which are not represented in trials [11].

These findings have informed the development of institutional pathways at centers such as MD Anderson Cancer Center, which integrate molecular test turnaround time, performance status, and comorbidity burden into treatment selection algorithms [12].

A parallel initiative in France, the ESME (Epidemiological Strategy and Medical Economics) platform, extracts structured oncology data from over 150 comprehensive cancer centers, enabling rapid comparative effectiveness studies. A landmark analysis of 20,446 women with metastatic breast cancer enrolled in the ESME cohort between 2008 and 2017 documented progressive improvements in overall survival across subtypes, coinciding with increasing uptake of CDK4/6 inhibitors from 2016 onwards - providing population-level confirmation that new treatment approvals were reaching and benefiting patients in routine practice [13].

Building on this, a target trial emulation study using 32,598 ESME patients successfully reproduced the findings of eight pivotal randomized trials, and demonstrated a statistically significant overall survival benefit with palbociclib (HR 0.81, 95% CI 0.72–0.92) that the original PALOMA-2 trial had been insufficiently powered to detect [14]. These findings illustrate how RWE from national oncology registries can both validate trial results and resolve uncertainties that controlled trials leave unanswered, directly informing treatment sequencing recommendations.

## 12.2. Integrated Care

Integrated care models - whether Accountable Care Organizations (ACOs) in the US, Integrated Care Systems (ICS) in England, or regional health cooperatives in the Netherlands - depend on RWE to align incentives, coordinate services, and track population-level outcomes. The adoption of HL7 FHIR application programming interfaces and nationally mandated shared care record infrastructures has provided the technical backbone for real-time, cross-institutional data exchange that makes such platforms operationally viable. Table 12.1 provides examples of integrated care dashboards and their impact.

**Table 12.1 Real World Applications of Integrated Care Dashboards**

| Region | Program | Data Sources Integrated | Primary Use Case | Reported Impact |
|---|---|---|---|---|
| **USA (PA)** | Geisinger ProvenCare | Claims, EHR, SDOH surveys | Risk stratification & intensive managemen t | 24% ↓ 30-day readmission s [11] |
| **UK (Greater Manchester)** | Salford ICP Dashboard | EMIS/SystmOn e, social care, remote monitoring | Real-time alerts for high-risk patients | 13% ↓ avoidable admissions [15] |
| **Nordic (DK/SE/NO)** | Nordic Health Data Platform | National disease, prescription, hospital registries | Cross-borde r comparative effectivenes s | 12% ↓ mortality in early HF Rx [13] |
| **USA (Midwest)** | CommonW ell Diabetes Registry | Multi-EHR, lab, imaging via FHIR | Eliminate duplicate testing & improve screening | 28% ↓ duplicate labs [18] |

## 12.2.1. Population Risk Stratification Across Care Settings

The Geisinger Health System in Pennsylvania built a ProvenCare analytics engine that combines claims, EHR, and social determinants of health (SDOH) data - including housing instability and food insecurity - to generate a composite care complexity score for each enrolled patient [15]. Patients in the highest risk decile receive intensified care management: home visits, medication reconciliation, and behavioral health outreach.

A multinational observational study using linked heart failure registries across Sweden, the United States, and the United Kingdom analyzed outcomes in patients initiating sacubitril/valsartan for heart failure with reduced ejection fraction, demonstrating that drug uptake rates, titration to target dose, and treatment continuity were each independently associated with all-cause mortality and hospitalization for heart failure over 18 months of follow-up [16]. These findings, integrated into updated ESC heart failure management guidelines [14], highlight how longitudinal registry-based RWE can directly shape prescribing recommendations across health systems.

An OECD review of integrated care analytics found that cross-sector RWE platforms reduce fragmentation and improve chronic disease outcomes, particularly when social care data are included [18].

Real-world cardiometabolic evidence has also reshaped population-level treatment strategies for patients with heart failure, obesity, and type 2 diabetes. Registry-based and large observational analyses have confirmed that SGLT2 inhibitors substantially reduce the risk of hospitalization for heart failure across populations far broader than those enrolled in landmark trials [19]- including patients with obesity, advanced chronic kidney disease, and multiple comorbidities.

Complementing these findings, the CVD-REAL program, a multinational analysis linking health databases and registries across six countries, demonstrated that patients initiated on SGLT2 inhibitors had significantly lower rates of hospitalization for heart failure and all-cause death compared with those started on other glucose-lowering agents, with consistent effects across diverse healthcare systems [20]. GLP-1 receptor agonist RWE has similarly expanded from cardiovascular risk reduction in type 2 diabetes to cardiorenal benefits in heart failure with preserved ejection fraction and obesity - findings that have prompted rapid updating of integrated care pathways for the treatment of cardiometabolic disease in several national guideline bodies.

### 12.2.2. Care Coordination Dashboards and Interoperability

The Coordinate My Care (CMC) program, developed at the Royal Marsden NHS Foundation Trust and commissioned as a pan-London NHS service, deployed a shared digital urgent care coordination platform accessible to GPs, community nurses, hospital clinicians, emergency department physicians, ambulance crews, NHS 111 providers, and social care workers across all five London Integrated Care Systems [20]. The platform consolidates patient-reported care preferences, ceiling-of-treatment decisions, resuscitation status, active medication records, and preferred place of care into a single, real-time digital care plan - visible to any authorized health or social care professional at the point of clinical contact, whether in a care home, an emergency department, or during an out-of-hours call, via integration with local EHR systems (EMIS, SystmOne, Cerner) and the London Care Record. By 2024, over 80,000 live care plans were in active use across 40 NHS trusts and 1,400 general practices, with more than 10,000 monthly accesses by urgent and emergency care staff alone.

A retrospective cohort analysis of 21,231 CMC patients who died between 2011 and 2019 found that those with a documented "not-for-resuscitation" status had a 57% lower likelihood of dying in hospital (OR 0.43; 95% CI 0.37–0.50), while the absence of any documented care preference was independently associated with a 43% higher probability of an acute hospital death compared with patients who had recorded their wishes [21].

A comparable US effort is the CommonWell Health Alliance, a not-for-profit health IT network that enables cross-organizational data sharing among >15 000 provider sites [22]. In a pilot across three Midwest health systems, CommonWell facilitated the creation of a shared registry of diabetic patients, integrating HbA1c measurements, retinal screening dates, and foot-exam records. Clinicians at any participating site could instantly view the latest comprehensive diabetes metrics, reducing duplicate testing by 28% and improving adherence to annual complication screenings [23].

## 12.3. Quality Improvement

Quality improvement (QI) initiatives increasingly rely on RWE to define baselines, detect variation, and sustain gains over time. Two complementary frameworks dominate:

- Audit-feedback cycles (e.g., national clinical audits)
- Continuous learning systems (e.g., Lean, Six Sigma, Plan-Do-Study-Act).

### 12.3.1. The Plan-Do-Study-Act Cycle with RWE

The Plan-Do-Study-Act (PDSA) cycle, demonstrated in

Figure 12.2 provides a systematic framework for continuous quality improvement using real-world evidence. It drives measurable change through iterative testing and learning.

- **Plan**: Establish baseline real-world evidence from routine practice. For example, 12 months of surgical site infection (SSI) surveillance might reveal an 8.5% infection rate, quantifying the problem and setting improvement targets.
- **Do**: Implement evidence-based interventions on a small scale. For example, an SSI prevention bundle including preoperative chlorhexidine washing, antibiotic prophylaxis, is introduced to minimize risk while identifying implementation barriers.
- **Study**: Analyze real-world data to evaluate impact, transforming data into actionable insights.
- **Act**: Decide whether to adopt and scale the intervention, adapt through another cycle, or abandon the approach.

Multiple sequential PDSA cycles build upon previous learning. Real-world evidence serves as both foundation and continuous feedback mechanism.

### 12.3.2. National Clinical Audits and Benchmarking

The UK National Clinical Audit and Patient Outcomes Programme (NCAPOP) publishes outcomes for over 40 conditions, ranging from hip fracture to cardiac surgery. Each audit links hospital data to national mortality and readmission databases, producing risk-adjusted performance metrics that are publicly reported [24].

The *Hip Fracture Audit*, for example, demonstrated that hospitals meeting the "golden hour" criterion - surgery within 36 hours of admission - had a five percentage point lower 30-day mortality compared with those falling below this threshold. Hospitals below the benchmark received targeted mentoring and process redesign support, resulting in a system-wide improvement from 68% to 86% compliance over four years [25].

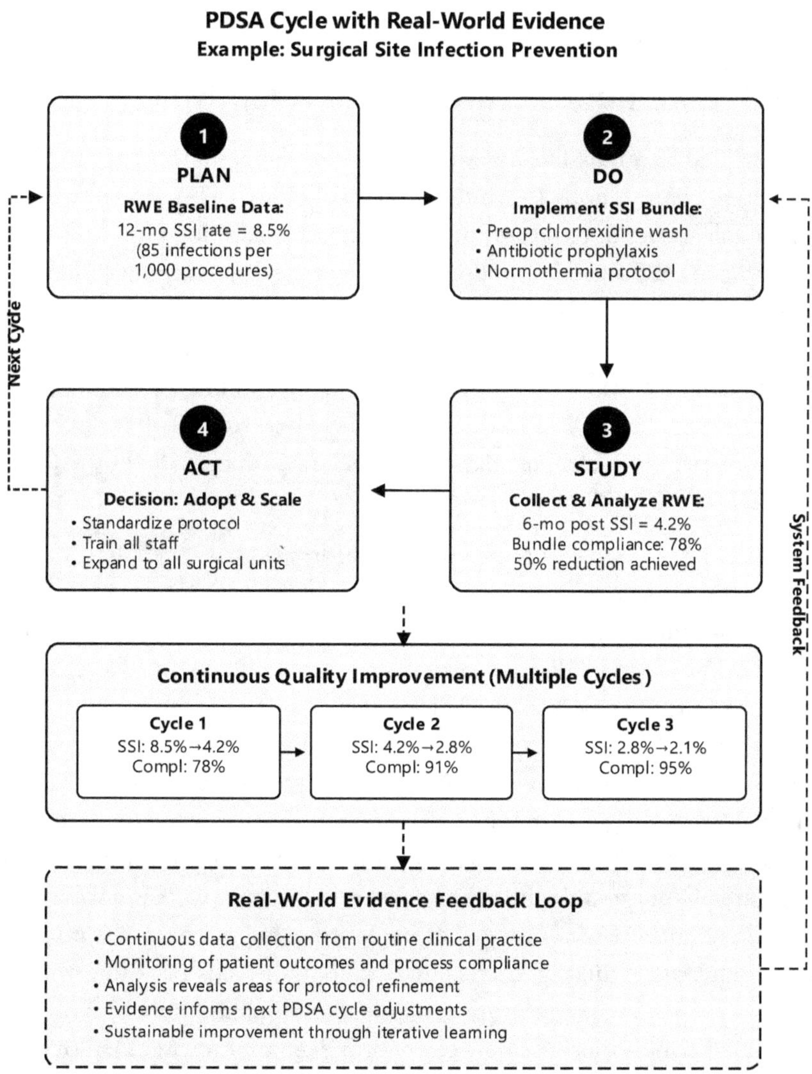


**Figure 12.2 Flow Diagram of a Plan-Do-Study-Act**

In the United States, the Society of Thoracic Surgeons (STS) National Database collects procedural detail, complications, and long-term follow-up for over 90% of cardiac operations [26]. Participating centers receive real-time dashboards comparing their observed-to-expected (O/E) mortality ratios. A multi-center QI project used STS data to identify variability in perioperative beta-blocker use; standardizing the protocol across 12 hospitals reduced 30-day major adverse cardiac events from 4.8% to 3.1% [27].

## 12.3.3. Continuous Learning and Adaptive QI

The Veterans Health Administration (VHA) in the US has pioneered a Continuous Learning Health System (CLHS) model, wherein every clinical encounter contributes to a national learning loop [28]. One flagship project focused on reducing catheter-associated urinary tract infections (CAUTI). Using national EHR data, the CLHS identified high-variation sites, deployed a bundle of evidence-based practices (e.g., daily catheter necessity assessment, aseptic insertion kits), and tracked CAUTI rates weekly. The CAUTI rates decreased from 2.40 to 2.05 infections per 1000 catheter-days (incidence rate ratio, 0.86; 95% CI, 0.76 to 0.96; P=0.009) [29].

Kaiser Permanente Northern California's Advance Alert Monitor (AAM) is the most rigorously evaluated example of RWD driving a continuous clinical learning loop. The system applies a machine learning model - trained on EHR data from over 1.5 million patients - to calculate an hourly deterioration risk score for every non-ICU inpatient, drawing on vital signs, laboratory results, severity-of-illness indices, comorbidity burden, and length-of-stay data. When a patient's score crosses the alert threshold, signaling an estimated risk of clinical deterioration within 12 hours of at least 8%, an automated notification is sent not to the bedside team directly but to a dedicated regional nursing hub, whose staff review the full patient record remotely before coordinating with on-site rapid response teams. Crucially, each clinical encounter feeds back into the system - performance monitoring, alert calibration, and nursing protocols are refined continuously as new real-world data accumulate. Deployed across 19 hospitals in a staggered stepped-wedge rollout between 2016 and 2019, the program was associated with a 16% relative reduction in 30-day mortality among alerted patients (adjusted RR 0.84; 95% CI 0.78-0.90) across nearly 550,000 hospitalizations [30].

## 12.4. Conclusion

RWE is proving indispensable for clinical and operational decision-making across the healthcare continuum. Within hospitals, it powers real-time decision support, optimizes antimicrobial and oncology pathways, and enhances patient safety. In integrated care systems, RWE enables cross-setting risk stratification, coordinated dashboards, and population health management - bridging primary, secondary, and social care. In quality improvement, both large-scale audit programs and continuous learning loops leverage RWE to set baselines, identify unwarranted variation, and sustain evidence-based practice changes.

What unites these applications is a shared methodological foundation: robust data curation, transparent analytic choices, and a commitment to contextual relevance - ensuring that the evidence generated reflects the patients and systems it seeks to serve. As interoperability standards mature (e.g., FHIR, OMOP CDM) and analytic tools become more embedded in clinical workflows, the boundary between "evidence generation" and "evidence use" will continue to blur, ushering in an era where every care episode contributes to - and benefits from - a learning health system.

### References

1. Henry KE, Hager DN, Pronovost PJ, et al. A targeted real-time early warning score (TREWScore) for septic shock. Sci Transl Med. 2015;7(299):299ra122.

2. Adams R, Henry KE, Sridharan A, et al. Prospective, multi-site study of patient outcomes after implementation of the TREWS machine learning-based early warning system for sepsis. Nat Med. 2022;28(7):1455–1460..

3. Shimabukuro DW, Barton CW, Feldman MD, et al. Effect of a machine learning-based severe sepsis prediction algorithm on patient survival and hospital length of stay: a randomised clinical trial. BMJ Open Respir Res. 2017;4(1):e000234.

4. Gerry S, Bonnici T, Birks J, et al. Early warning scores for detecting deterioration in adult hospital patients: systematic review and critical appraisal of methodology. BMJ. 2020;369:m1501.

5. van de Klundert N, Holman R, Dongelmans DA, et al. Data resource profile: the Dutch National Intensive Care Evaluation (NICE) registry of admissions to adult intensive care units. Int J Epidemiol. 2015;44(6):1850–1850h.

6. Obermeyer Z, Powers B, Vogeli C, et al. Dissecting racial bias in an algorithm used to manage the health of populations. Science. 2019;366(6464):447-453.

7. Labkoff S, Oladimeji B, Kannry J, et al. Toward a responsible future: recommendations for AI-enabled clinical decision support. J Am Med Inform Assoc. 2024;31(11):2730–2739.

8. CDC. Antibiotic Resistance Laboratory Network (AR Lab Network). 2025.

9. Royal College of General Practitioners (RCGP). TARGET Antibiotics Toolkit. 2023.

10. UK Health Security Agency. English Surveillance Programme for Antimicrobial Utilisation and Resistance (ESPAUR) Report 2022 to 2023. London: UKHSA; 2023.

11. Khozin S, Abernethy AP, Nussbaum NC, et al. Characteristics of real-world metastatic non-small cell lung cancer patients treated with nivolumab and pembrolizumab during the year following approval. Oncologist. 2018;23(3):328-336.

12. MD Anderson Cancer Center. NSCLC Treatment Pathway v3.1. Houston, TX: MD Anderson Cancer Center; 2024.

13. Grinda T, Antoine A, Jacot W, et al. Evolution of overall survival and receipt of new therapies by subtype among 20 446 metastatic breast cancer patients in the 2008-2017 ESME cohort. ESMO Open. 2021;6(3):100114.

14. Antoine A, Pérol D, Robain M, et al. Assessing the real-world effectiveness of 8 major metastatic breast cancer drugs using target trial emulation. Eur J Cancer. 2024 Dec;213:115072.

15. Steele GD, Haynes JA, Davis DE, et al. How Geisinger's advanced medical home model argues the case for rapid-cycle innovation. Health Aff (Millwood). 2010;29(11):2047–2053.

16. Savarese G, Bodegård J, Norhammar A, et al. Heart failure drug titration, discontinuation, mortality and heart failure hospitalisations: a multinational observational study (US, Sweden, and UK). Eur J Heart Fail. 2021;23(9):1499–1511.

17. McDonagh TA, Metra M, Adamo M, et al. 2021 ESC Guidelines for the diagnosis and treatment of acute and chronic heart failure. Eur Heart J. 2021;42(36):3599–3726.

18. OECD. Realising the Potential of Primary Health Care. Paris: OECD Publishing; 2020.

19. Kosiborod MN, Abildstrøm SZ, Borlaug BA, et al. Semaglutide in patients with heart failure with preserved ejection fraction and obesity. N Engl J Med. 2023;389(12):1069–1084.

20. Callender T, Riley J, Broadhurst HL, et al. The determinants of dying where we choose: an analysis of Coordinate My Care. Ann Intern Med. 2017;167(7):519–521.

21. Orlovic M, Callender T, Riley J, et al. Impact of advance care planning on dying in hospital: evidence from urgent care records. PLoS One. 2020;15(12):e0242914.

22. CommonWell Health Alliance. 2025 Annual Report. https://commonwellalliance.org/annual-report-2025/

23. Patel V, et al. Cross-EHR diabetes registry reduces duplicate testing and improves screening adherence: a Midwest health system pilot. Health Aff (Millwood). 2024;43(7):978–987.

24. NHS England. National Clinical Audit and Patient Outcomes Programme. 2025. https://www.nhs.uk/audits/

25. Royal College of Physicians. Hip Fracture Audit Quality Improvement Programme. 2025 update.

26. Society of Thoracic Surgeons. STS National Database Annual Report 2024. Chicago: STS.

27. Brennan JM, et al. Standardising perioperative beta-blocker use across 12 cardiac surgery centres: a multi-institutional QI initiative. Ann Thorac Surg. 2023;115(4):1152–1160.

28. Department of Veterans Affairs. Continuous Learning Health System (CLHS) Blueprint. 2024.

29. Saint S, Greene MT, Krein SL, et al. A program to prevent catheter-associated urinary tract infection in acute care. N Engl J Med. 2016;374(22):2111–2119.

30. Escobar GJ, Liu VX, Schuler A, et al. Automated identification of adults at risk for in-hospital clinical deterioration. N Engl J Med. 2020;383(20):1951–1960.

# Chapter 13. RWE in Pharma and Life Sciences

The pharmaceutical and life sciences industry has long relied on randomized controlled trials (RCTs) to establish the safety and efficacy of new therapies. However, as healthcare systems demand more evidence on how treatments perform in routine clinical practice, real-world evidence (RWE) has become an indispensable complement to traditional clinical development. RWE enables biopharmaceutical companies to address questions that cannot be answered in the highly controlled context of registration trials - questions about long-term safety, comparative effectiveness across heterogeneous populations, economic value, and post-market performance.

By 2026, the maturity of federated data networks and the formalization of global regulatory frameworks have moved RWE from a "supportive" role to a "core" requirement for initial market entry and sustained reimbursement.

This chapter outlines how RWE is operationalized across four core pillars of pharma activity: safety surveillance, effectiveness research, market access, health economics and outcomes research (HEOR), and commercial performance. Each section highlights methodological considerations, regulatory expectations, and concrete global examples - illustrating how RWE strengthens decision-making from early development through lifecycle management. The emphasis remains on practical application: how RWE studies are conceived, executed, and integrated into strategic functions while meeting the evidentiary standards of regulators, payers, and clinicians.

## 13.1. Safety

Although clinical trials provide initial safety signals, they are rarely powered to detect rare or delayed adverse events. The International Council for Harmonisation (ICH) E2E guideline underscores the need for proactive risk management supported by real-world data (RWD) post-approval [1]. In practice, pharmacovigilance in the life sciences industry has evolved from passive spontaneous reporting to active, data-driven surveillance using large-scale RWD sources.

Large healthcare databases - such as the US FDA's Sentinel System, the EU's EudraVigilance Data Analysis System (EVDAS), and Japan's Medical Information Database Center (JMDC) - enable near real-time safety monitoring. Table 13.1 summarizes key RWD/RWE sources used globally for safety surveillance, with their structural strengths and limitations.

A notable example is the FDA's use of Sentinel to evaluate the risk of angioedema with angiotensin receptor-neprilysin inhibitors (ARNIs), comparing sacubitril/valsartan to angiotensin convertor enzyme (ACE) inhibitors and angiotensin receptor blockers in approximately 70,000 matched heart failure patients. The analysis found no increased risk of angioedema among de novo sacubitril/valsartan initiators compared with new users of either drug class, while identifying an elevated risk in patients who recently switched from prior ACE inhibitor therapy - a finding with direct implications for clinical guidance on transition protocols [2]. The FDA Sentinel System has since expanded its active safety surveillance capabilities, including the development of natural language processing approaches to analyze unstructured clinician notes, with the aim of improving detection of adverse events that are otherwise under-coded in structured claims data [3].

**Table 13.1 Global RWD Sources for Pharmacovigilance**

| Region | Source | Coverage | Key Strengths | Limitations |
|---|---|---|---|---|
| **United States** | FDA Sentinel (CMS, Optum, IBM MarketScan) | ~300 million patients | Near real-time; modular analytic infrastructure | Limited clinical detail; variable coding quality |
| **European Union** | EMA's DARWIN EU | >150 million (+16 countries) | Centralized federated analysis; OMOP CDM | Heterogeneous coding; fragmented access |
| **Japan** | JMDC Claims & EMR Database | ~7 million | Linkable claims + EMR; longitudinal | Not nationally representative; limited elderly coverage |
| **Canada** | CNODES (Canadian Network for Observational Drug Effect Studies) | ~50 million (provincial linkage) | Population-based; validated algorithms | Delays in data availability (~2 years) |

In Europe, the PROTECT consortium demonstrated how distributed data networks, such as the EU-ADR and OMOP platforms, can harmonize heterogeneous national databases to conduct multinational safety studies - e.g., quantifying the risk of upper gastrointestinal bleeding with NSAIDs across five countries [4].

A critical challenge lies in distinguishing true signals from confounding-by-indication. Consider a hypothetical safety query: Does Drug X increase the risk of acute kidney injury (AKI)? In real-life, patients prescribed Drug X are often sicker, with more comorbidities and polypharmacy - factors independently associated with AKI. Advanced methods (e.g., high-dimensional propensity score adjustment, self-controlled case series) are now routinely embedded in safety protocols to mitigate such bias [4].

Alongside database-driven pharmacovigilance, spontaneous reporting systems continue to serve a complementary role through disproportionality analysis. Methods such as the reporting odds ratio (ROR) and information component (IC) applied to national and international repositories - including the FDA Adverse Event Reporting System (FAERS) and the WHO VigiBase - provide rapid hypothesis generation at scale, particularly for newly approved agents where database exposure is still limited. Combining disproportionality signals with confirmatory analyses in structured RWD databases represents best practice in contemporary pharmacovigilance programs.

## 13.2. Effectiveness

While RCTs answer "Can this drug work under ideal conditions?", RWE addresses "Does it work in everyday practice, for whom, and under what circumstances?" Effectiveness studies are increasingly embedded in regulatory post-approval requirements (e.g., FDA's post-marketing commitments) and used internally for lifecycle management - such as supporting new indications, dosage forms, or combination therapies. Box 13.1 lists typical use cases of RWE in effectiveness research.

**Box 13.1 Typical Use Cases for RWE in Effectiveness Research**

1. Supporting label expansions (e.g., new line of therapy, broader age range)
2. Generating external control arms for single-arm trials (e.g., in rare diseases)
3. Assessing durability of response beyond trial follow-up (e.g., 5-year survival in immuno-oncology)
4. Evaluating effectiveness in underrepresented subgroups (e.g., pregnant women, frail elderly)
5. Informing clinical pathway adoption by health systems

A prominent example is the use of RWE to support the 2020 FDA approval of pembrolizumab for tumor mutational burden-high (TMB-H) solid tumors. Although the pivotal KEYNOTE-158 trial was prospective, complementary whole-exome sequencing analyses from multiple pembrolizumab clinical trials - encompassing several thousand additional patients across diverse tumor types - reinforced confidence in

TMB-H as a pan-tumor predictive biomarker, ultimately informing the FDA's decision to grant accelerated approval [6].

In Europe, Roche leveraged the Danish National Patient Registry and Danish Cancer Registry to demonstrate that trastuzumab emtansine (T-DM1) improved progression-free survival vs. lapatinib + capecitabine in HER2+ metastatic breast cancer patients ineligible for clinical trials - providing external validity to the EMILIA trial results [7].

Effectiveness studies often compare active treatments (rather than placebo), necessitating careful control of confounding. Propensity score matching (PSM), inverse probability weighting (IPW), and targeted maximum likelihood estimation (TMLE) are now standard in pharma-sponsored studies. For instance, in the CVD-REAL study comparing SGLT2 inhibitors versus other glucose-lowering drugs for cardiovascular outcomes, AstraZeneca-funded investigators used propensity score matching and a new-user design across multinational databases from six countries (the United States, Germany, Sweden, Norway, Denmark, and the United Kingdom) to emulate a target trial, demonstrating lower risk of heart failure hospitalization and all-cause death with SGLT2 inhibitor initiation - a finding consistent across countries and glucose-lowering drug comparators [8].

Crucially, effectiveness is not synonymous with "lower efficacy." Rather, it reflects contextual performance - including adherence, dosing patterns, concomitant medications, and disease severity. A well-designed RWE effectiveness study should therefore specify:

- The **target trial emulation** framework (Hernán & Robins, 2016) [9]
- The **population of interest** (e.g., elderly, renal-impaired, polypharmacy)
- The comparator(s) aligned with standard of care in relevant geographies

## 13.3. Market Access

Payers - whether national health services (e.g., NHS England, Germany's G-BA), private insurers (e.g., UnitedHealth, AXA), or managed care organizations - require evidence not only of clinical benefit but of comparative value. As discussed thoroughly in Chapter 11. RWE plays a pivotal role in health technology assessment (HTA), especially when RCTs lack head-to-head comparisons, long-term outcomes, or cost-related endpoints.

In the US, the Institute for Clinical and Economic Review (ICER) routinely incorporates RWE in its value assessments. For example, in its 2022 review of inclisiran for hypercholesterolemia, ICER supplemented trial data with a Markov model calibrated using real-world LDL-C trajectories from the UK Clinical Practice Research Datalink (CPRD), estimating long-term cardiovascular event reductions over 30 years [10].

In Europe, the French Haute Autorité de Santé (HAS) explicitly encourages RWE in *Amélioration du Service Médical Rendu* (ASMR – improvement of the provided medical service) dossiers when RCTs are insufficient - e.g., for orphan drugs where trial size is constrained. The landscape of market access was fundamentally reshaped in 2025 by the implementation of the EU Health Technology Assessment Regulation (EUHTAR). This regulation mandates "Joint Clinical Assessments" (JCA) for all new oncology drugs and Advanced Therapy Medicinal Products (ATMPs) across the EU. Under this framework, RWE is now explicitly used to bridge gaps in comparative effectiveness between the new therapy and the "standard of care" in different member states [11].

A distinctive feature of market access RWE is its geographic specificity. A study supporting reimbursement in Italy must reflect Italian practice patterns, formulary constraints, and coding conventions. Novartis' submission of secukinumab for ankylosing spondylitis in Spain included a retrospective cohort study using the Spanish EpiChron cohort, demonstrating real-world drug survival rates >80% at 12 months - addressing payer concerns about early discontinuation [12].

Similarly, in emerging markets, RWE can substitute for local trials: in Brazil, ANVISA accepted a study using the DATASUS public health database to support biosimilar infliximab uptake, citing comparable hospitalization rates vs. originator [13].

Methodologically, market access studies increasingly integrate hybrid designs - e.g., pragmatic trials embedded in routine care (like the ADAPTABLE trial of aspirin dosing [14]) or prospective registries with embedded economic endpoints (e.g., the German AQUA registry for cardiac devices). For orphan drugs, the use of "Synthetic Control Arms" (SCAs) has moved from experimental to expected; multiple payers accepted SCAs as a valid comparison for single-arm trials in rare genetic disorders [15].

## 13.4. Health Economics and Outcomes Research (HEOR)

HEOR is where RWE converges with patient-centeredness, economic modeling, and quality measurement.

In pharma, HEOR teams use RWD to quantify:

- **Resource utilization:** hospitalizations, ER visits, outpatient visits,
- **Productivity loss:** absenteeism, presenteeism (often via PRO-linked databases like NHANES or national workforce surveys),
- **Patient-reported outcomes (PROs):** symptom burden, quality of life, treatment satisfaction.

A landmark example is the cost-effectiveness analysis of hepatitis C direct-acting antivirals (DAAs). Using a decision-analytic Markov model parameterized with clinical trial efficacy data and real-world cost inputs, the investigators estimated lifetime costs and quality-adjusted life years (QALYs) for sofosbuvir/ledipasvir treatment in the United States, demonstrating that - even at the list price of approximately $95,000 per treatment course - DAA therapy was cost-effective at conventional willingness-to-pay thresholds when accounting for avoided cirrhosis progression and hepatocellular carcinoma [16].

In Europe, the EQ-5D index derived from routine EHRs is gaining traction. In Sweden, Karolinska Institutet and AstraZeneca collaborated on a study using the Stockholm-Gotland registry to map real-world EQ-5D trajectories in COPD patients initiating triple therapy - revealing meaningful improvements ($\Delta$EQ-5D $\geq$0.07) sustained over 24 months, supporting premium pricing negotiations [17].

Table 13.2 presents common RWE endpoints and PROs.

**Table 13.2 Common RWE Endpoints in HEOR Studies by Therapeutic Area**

| Therapeutic Area | Clinical Endpoint | Economic Endpoint | PRO Endpoint | Typical Data Sources |
|---|---|---|---|---|
| **Cardiovascular** | MACE, HF hospitalization | 30-day readmission cost | KCCQ, EQ-5D | CMS, CPRD, SWEDEHEART |
| **Oncology** | OS, PFS, treatment lines | Cost per line, supportive care use | EORTC QLQ-C30, PROMIS | Flatiron, SEER-Medicare, NCR |
| **Rare diseases** | Disease progression (clinician-assessed) | Lifetime care cost modeling | PedsQL, SF-36 | RD-Connect, EURORDIS registries |
| **CNS (e.g., MS)** | Relapse rate, EDSS change | DMT switch cost, MRI utilization | MSIS-29, NARCOMS | MSBase, Swedish MS Registry |

MACE = major adverse cardiac events; HF = heart failure; OS = overall survival; PFS = progression-free survival; DMT = disease-modifying therapy; EDSS = Expanded Disability Status Scale.

PROs remain challenging in claims/EHR data, but hybrid collection is emerging. The FDA's Project Optimus encourages sponsors to optimize dosing in oncology, with growing emphasis on integrating patient-reported outcome measures into dose-finding studies to capture tolerability alongside efficacy. Pfizer's PROmpt initiative embedded a 5-item fatigue scale in the Epic EHR for breast cancer patients, identifying subgroups with disproportionate symptom burden - enabling targeted supportive care interventions [18]. Whenever available, tokenization of patient data allows connecting prospectively collected PROs to retrospective HER and registries.

When modeling budget impact, pharma teams now link clinical RWE outcomes to local cost data (e.g., DRG weights, outpatient tariffs), improving realism over hypothetical assumptions.

## 13.5. Commercial Analytics & Brand Performance

Beyond its roles in safety, effectiveness, market access, and HEOR, RWE has become a foundational instrument for the commercial functions of pharmaceutical companies. We expand this section as compared to other topics, as it is not discussed elsewhere in this book. Also, the volume of "studies" and "reports" generated for commercial purposes in pharma is probably equal if not greater than all other forms of real-world studies produced for regulators and payers combined. Finally, it is to be noted that the commercial use of RWD historically started before its scientific use. The first systems of organized EHR data collection such as the ancestors of CPRD and IQVIA Xponent, started in 1980s for commercial purposes. Methodologically, some of the analytical and data science methods applied for commercial use of RWD are scientifically and computationally ahead of those used in epidemiology and statistics, albeit invisible to the scientific community as often not published.

While the preceding sections address questions primarily of clinical or economic relevance to external stakeholders - regulators, payers, and clinicians - commercial teams use RWD to answer an equally demanding set of questions: Who is prescribing our product, and to which patients? How does observed market share compare with the addressable treatment population? Where and why are patients discontinuing, switching, or never initiating therapy? These questions are operational in nature but carry direct implications for revenue trajectory, brand lifecycle management, and strategic resource allocation. Box 13.2 summarizes the principal use cases in which commercial teams deploy RWD analytics.

### 13.5.1. Prescribing activity

The most foundational commercial application of RWD is the measurement of prescribing activity and market share. Prescription audit databases - such as the IQVIA Xponent and MIDAS platforms, or Symphony Health's longitudinal claims dataset covering more than 300 million US patients - provide near real-time tracking of total and new prescriptions (TRx and NRx) at the level of individual prescribers, geographic regions, and payer channels [19]. These data allow commercial teams to benchmark brand performance against competitors, monitor the impact of promotional interventions, identify geographic pockets of underutilization, and calibrate field force deployment.

In the European context, dispensing data from national health registries (e.g., the NHS Business Services Authority in England, the GKV Datentransparenz in Germany, or the SNDS in France) serve analogous functions, albeit with varying levels of prescriber-level granularity and access lag. In some cases, the access is not allowed for studies which cannot show public interest.

### 13.5.2. Treatment pathways

A second and increasingly strategically important domain is the analysis of treatment pathways and patient journey dynamics. Using longitudinal patient-level claims or EHR data, commercial and medical affairs teams can reconstruct sequences of therapy - from the point of diagnosis through multiple lines of treatment - at population scale. Metrics such as time to treatment initiation, duration of therapy, persistence rates, and source of business (i.e., the proportion of new prescriptions attributable to de novo initiators versus patients switching from a competitor) provide granular intelligence that aggregate market share figures cannot offer [19].

In multiple sclerosis, for example, analysis of treatment sequences across more than 14,000 patients in the US IBM MarketScan database revealed over 400 distinct DMT pathway patterns and showed that approximately 70% of patients switched or discontinued their initial therapy within two years - insights of direct relevance to both brand positioning and patient support program design [20]. Analogous analyses in oncology, rheumatology, and cardiometabolic disease have demonstrated that the gap between guideline-recommended and real-world treatment uptake is often substantial, creating identifiable commercial opportunities as well as clinical quality concerns.

The analysis of treatment discontinuation and switching deserves particular attention, as it is one of the areas where commercial and medical interests most naturally converge. Retrospective database studies, when enriched with unstructured clinical notes analyzed using natural language processing, can move beyond the binary observation that a patient stopped therapy to reveal the clinically documented reasons - tolerability issues, formulary barriers, lack of perceived benefit, or prescriber preference for an alternative [19]. McKinsey estimates that an average top-20 pharmaceutical company could unlock more than $300 million per year in commercial value by systematically deploying advanced RWE analytics across its in-market and pipeline portfolio, with switch and discontinuation analytics representing among the highest-value use cases [21]. Understanding the drivers of discontinuation is not merely a commercial exercise: it identifies unmet needs that can guide investment in patient support programs, dosing optimization studies, or next-generation formulations.

## 13.5.3. Adherence and persistence

A further use case lies in adherence and persistence monitoring. Administrative claims data permit calculation of medication possession ratios (MPR) and proportion of days covered (PDC) at scale, enabling commercial teams to stratify patients by adherence profile and identify subpopulations at elevated risk of dropout. These insights directly feed into patient services strategy - for example, determining which patient cohorts benefit most from specialty pharmacy intervention, copay assistance programs, or nurse navigator support.

For example, in a real-world study of GLP-1 receptor agonists, dulaglutide demonstrated significantly higher 12-month persistence than weekly semaglutide or exenatide across commercially insured patients in the United States - a finding of commercial as well as clinical relevance that influenced both brand messaging and patient support infrastructure [19].

### 13.5.4. Methodological considerations

Several methodological distinctions separate commercial RWD analytics from their clinical counterparts. The primary currency of commercial analytics is typically aggregated projected prescribing volume rather than individual-level patient outcomes; inferential causal claims are generally not the objective, and descriptive rigor - accurate patient counting, appropriate cohort definitions, and consistent treatment of combination therapies - is the dominant methodological concern.

A recurring challenge is the variable coverage of specialty pharmacy channels and hospital administration in standard prescription audit databases, which can lead to systematic underestimation of market size in oncology, rare disease, and biologics segments where dispensing occurs outside the retail pharmacy. Linking multiple data sources - retail Rx data, specialty pharmacy feeds, and medical claims - is therefore often necessary for a complete commercial picture [19].

### 13.5.5. Governance and compliance

Governance and compliance considerations also differentiate commercial from scientific RWE activities. Data used to inform field force targeting or promotional messaging must be handled under strict privacy frameworks - HIPAA in the United States, the GDPR in Europe - and any evidence used in external-facing communications with HCPs or payers must meet applicable promotional regulations and, increasingly, the evidentiary standards expected by medical affairs and regulatory affairs functions.

As the boundary between commercial and medical evidence generation continues to blur - with the same longitudinal datasets informing both brand strategy and post-approval regulatory commitments - leading companies are establishing integrated evidence governance frameworks that coordinate commercial, medical, HEOR, and pharmacovigilance teams around a common data infrastructure and methodological standards [21].

# 13.6. Conclusion

Real-world evidence has matured from an exploratory tool to a strategic asset across the pharmaceutical value chain. In safety, it enables proactive, scalable pharmacovigilance that complements spontaneous reporting. In effectiveness, it validates trial findings in broader populations and supports label evolution. In market access, it tailors evidence to payer priorities across diverse healthcare systems. In HEOR, it quantifies holistic value - clinical, economic, and humanistic - essential for sustainable pricing and reimbursement. In commercial, it allows understanding of the performance of the assets in real-world, as compared to their competitors, understand prescribing patterns, patient satisfaction and use.

Yet challenges persist: data fragmentation, methodological heterogeneity, and variable regulatory acceptance across regions. The industry's response has been threefold: (1) investment in standardized data platforms; (2) adoption of rigorous study designs (e.g., target trial emulation, active comparator new-user); and (3) early engagement with regulators and HTA bodies through scientific advice procedures.

As RWE becomes embedded in regulatory pathways - exemplified by FDA's RWE Framework (2018) [22], EMA's Big Data Steering Group outputs [23], and WHO's recent guidance on RWD for HTA [18] - pharma companies must ensure their RWE programs are fit-for-purpose, transparent, and ethically grounded. The future lies not in RWE replacing RCTs, but in a continuous evidence ecosystem where randomized and observational insights inform each other iteratively - ultimately delivering on the promise of precision, value-based, and patient-centered care.

## References

1. International Council for Harmonisation. ICH E2E: Pharmacovigilance planning. 2004.

2. Eworuke E, Welch EC, Haug N, et al. Comparative Risk of Angioedema With Sacubitril-Valsartan vs Renin-Angiotensin-Aldosterone Inhibitors. J Am Coll Cardiol. 2023;81(4):321–331.

3. US Food and Drug Administration. Sentinel System Five-Year Strategy 2019–2023. Silver Spring, MD: FDA; 2019.

4. Sturkenboom MC, Reynolds R, van Staa TP, et al. The PROTECT project: methodological development and practical implementation of distributed analyses for drug safety. Pharmacoepidemiol Drug Saf. 2013;22(S1):71–72.

5. Schneeweiss S. A basic study design for expedited safety signal evaluation based on electronic healthcare data. Pharmacoepidemiol Drug Saf. 2010 Aug;19(8):858–868.

6. Marcus L, Fashoyin-Aje LA, Donoghue M, et al. FDA Approval Summary: Pembrolizumab for the Treatment of Tumor Mutational Burden-High Solid Tumors. Clin Cancer Res. 2021;27(17):4685–4689.

7. Andersen SE, Jensen BV, Lajer H, et al. Real-world effectiveness of T-DM1 in HER2-positive metastatic breast cancer: a Danish nationwide cohort study. Breast Cancer Res Treat. 2020;184(2):477–487.

8. Kosiborod M, Cavender MA, Fu AZ, et al. Lower risk of heart failure and death in patients initiated on sodium-glucose cotransporter-2 inhibitors versus other glucose-lowering drugs: the CVD-REAL study (Comparative Effectiveness of Cardiovascular Outcomes in New Users of SGLT-2 Inhibitors). Circulation. 2017;136(3):249–259.

9. Hernán MA, Robins JM. Using big data to emulate a target trial when randomized trials are not available. Am J Epidemiol. 2016;183(8):758–764.

10. Institute for Clinical and Economic Review. Inclisiran for prevention of cardiovascular events: effectiveness and value. ICER Report. 2022.

11. European Commission. Regulation (EU) 2021/2282 on HTA: Implementation of Joint Clinical Assessments. Updated Jan 2025.

12. Gratacós J, Abásolo L, Alperi M, et al. Drug survival of secukinumab in ankylosing spondylitis: data from the Spanish EpiChron cohort. Rheumatology (Oxford). 2021;60(7):3310–3317.

13. Costa FA, Caetano R, Ferraz MB. Real-world effectiveness of biosimilar infliximab in Brazil: a retrospective cohort study using DATASUS. Value Health Reg Issues. 2020;22:105–111.

14. Jones WS, Mulder H, Wruck LM, et al. Comparative effectiveness of aspirin dosing in cardiovascular disease. N Engl J Med. 2021;384(21):1981–1990.

15. Garrison LP, et al. Using Synthetic Control Arms for HTA: A 2025 Consensus Report. Value Health. 2025;28(3):289-301.

16. Chhatwal J, Kanwal F, Roberts MS, et al. Cost-effectiveness and budget impact of hepatitis C virus treatment with sofosbuvir and ledipasvir in the United States. Ann Intern Med. 2015;162(6):397–406.

17. Jansson SA, Backman H, Rönmark E, et al. Real-world health-related quality of life in COPD patients treated with triple therapy: a Swedish registry-based study. Int J Chron Obstruct Pulmon Dis. 2022;17:1289–1300.

18. Basch E, Deal AM, Kris MG, et al. Symptom monitoring with patient-reported outcomes to enhance cancer care: the PROmpt trial. J Clin Oncol. 2023;41(16_suppl):TPS103.

19. Dagenais S, Russo L, Madsen A, et al. Use of real-world evidence to drive drug development strategy and inform clinical trial design. Clin Pharmacol Ther. 2022;111(1):77–89.

20. Xiao H, Princic M, Valle D, et al. Real-world disease-modifying therapy pathways from administrative claims data in patients with multiple sclerosis. BMC Neurol. 2022;22(1):218.

21. Anagnostopoulos C, Champagne D, Devereson A, et al. Generating real-world evidence at scale using advanced analytics. McKinsey Life Sciences Practice Report. McKinsey & Company; March 2022.

22. US Food and Drug Administration. Framework for FDA's Real-World Evidence Program. 2018.

23. European Medicines Agency. Big Data Steering Group: Work plan and deliverables. EMA/274129/2022.

24. World Health Organization. Using real-world data for health technology assessment: a global guidance framework. WHO Technical Series. 2023.

# Chapter 14. Real-World Evidence Strategy Planning

Real-world evidence generation is often reactive: a data asset becomes available (e.g., a new EHR partnership), a regulatory letter requests a post-marketing study, or a medical affairs team seeks market insights - and a study is launched. While technically feasible, such ad hoc approaches risk producing evidence that is **methodologically sound but strategically misaligned**: rigorous yet irrelevant to the intended decision-maker.

A new paradigm has already emerged: **evidence strategy planning** - the systematic, prospective design of an integrated evidence generation plan that spans the entire product lifecycle, anchored in stakeholder decision contexts, and optimized for fitness-for-purpose [1]. This approach treats evidence not as a deliverable, but as a strategic asset: dynamic, iterative, and purpose-built.

The FDA and EMA guidance on real-world evidence provide foundational methodological principles for conducting and assessing non-interventional studies (NIS) using RWD throughout a medicine's lifecycle [1,2]. They underscore the importance of pre-specified protocols, fit-for-purpose data sources, and transparent governance - core pillars of any evidence strategy.

This chapter operationalizes evidence strategy planning through three interlocking layers:

- **Lifecycle phase** (when is the evidence needed?),
- **Stakeholder evidence need** (what question must be answered?),
- **Fit-for-purpose pairing** (which design + data source achieves optimal validity and acceptability?)

## 14.1. Evidence Needs Across the Product Lifecycle

Real-world evidence is not a static deliverable - it evolves in purpose, design, and priority as a health technology progresses from target validation to post-generic sustainability. Each lifecycle phase presents distinct evidence gaps that RWE can - and increasingly must - address, often serving as the sole feasible or ethical route to answer high-stakes questions. Understanding this temporal dimension prevents misallocation of resources (e.g., launching a 5-year registry pre-Phase I) and ensures continuity: insights from early development inform post-approval commitments, and post-marketing learnings feed into next-generation innovation.

We organize evidence needs into five phases, aligned with regulatory, HTA, and commercial decision points, drawing on documented precedents of RWE use in submissions, approvals, and policy.

### 14.1.1. Pre-Approval

This phase starts with target identification and ends with regulatory submission. Before pivotal trials begin, RWE shapes feasibility, population selection, and comparator choice. The goal is to justify development, optimize trial design, and demonstrate unmet need.

Key needs include:

- **Disease epidemiology and natural history**: Critical for sample size calculation, site selection, and defining endpoints, especially in rare diseases where RCTs are impractical.

  Example: For tofersen, an antisense therapy for SOD1-ALS, Biogen used data from the Project MinE genomic registry and the U.S. National ALS Registry to characterize SOD1 mutation prevalence, estimated at approximately 2% of all ALS cases, supporting enrichment strategies and informing the design of the Phase III VALOR trial [4,5]. This natural history evidence was instrumental in justifying the trial's focus on a genetically defined subpopulation where traditional recruitment would have taken over a decade.

- **Standard of care (SoC) mapping**: Real-world treatment sequencing informs trial comparators and eligibility criteria.

  Example: In developing sotorasib for KRAS G12C-mutant NSCLC, Amgen analyzed Flatiron Health EHR data to demonstrate that a substantial proportion of patients with KRAS G12C-mutant disease received only one prior line of systemic therapy before further progression, informing the CodeBreaK 100 eligibility criterion of at least one prior systemic treatment and broadening the potential treatable population [6].

- **Burden of illness**: Required by HTA bodies to quantify unmet need, especially for ultra-orphan drugs.

  Example: For vutrisiran (ATTR amyloidosis), Alnylam submitted a burden-of-illness study combining THAOS registry data (disease progression), U.S. Medicare claims (hospitalisation costs), and patient interviews (QoL impact). This multi-source evidence (fitness A) was pivotal in EMA's 2022 approval and subsequent NICE appraisal [7].

- **Real-world trial eligibility**: EHR-based simulations routinely reveal poor external validity of RCT criteria.

Example: Multiple studies using real-world cancer registry and EHR data have documented that a substantial proportion of real-world patients with advanced solid tumors fail to meet eligibility for pivotal clinical trials - primarily due to comorbidities, organ dysfunction thresholds, and prior therapy requirements excluded in protocols [8]. Such insights now routinely trigger protocol broadening.

### 14.1.2. Peri-Approval

This phase spans from regulatory decision to commercial launch. At launch, RWE shifts toward system readiness and predictive validity - often shaping early access program (EAPs) and risk-sharing agreements. The goal is to support approval, prepare for reimbursement, and anticipate implementation.

The evidence needs include:

- **Budget impact forecasting**: Requires short-term uptake and cost models, calibrated with early real-world data.

  Example: For lecanemab (Alzheimer's disease), Eisai used IQVIA claims data from the U.S. Open-Label Extension and CLARITY AD RCT to model 3-year uptake and infusion costs. HAS required this to estimate annual budget impact - leading to a phased rollout with mandatory RWE monitoring [9].

- **Indication-specific epidemiology**: Narrowed prevalence to the approved population - critical for orphan drugs.

  Example: For elranatamab (BCMA+ relapsed/refractory myeloma), Pfizer combined Flatiron EHR, SEER cancer registry, and Medicare claims to estimate U.S. prevalence at 2,800 patients - directly informing FDA's Breakthrough Therapy designation and CMS coverage with evidence development (CED) criteria [8].

- **Risk minimization measures**: Can risk evaluation and mitigation (REMS) or risk minimization measures (RMMs) be implemented? Chart reviews and workflow assessments identify barriers early.

Example: Prior to tisagenlecleucel's EU launch, Novartis conducted EHR chart reviews across 12 CAR-T centres to assess apheresis-to-infusion timelines. Findings revealed median 28-day delays (vs. 21-day trial window), prompting revised logistics and staff training - later validated in the ELIANA real-world cohort [10].

### 14.1.3. Early Post-Approval

This phase encompasses the first three years post launch. The first post-approval years are high-stakes: regulators mandate PASS/PAES, payers negotiate outcomes-based contracts, and clinicians seek real-world guidance. The goal is to fulfill regulatory commitments, demonstrate real-world value, and optimize uptake.

The needs include:

- **Drug utilisation studies (DUS)**: Regulators could mandate DUS for all new molecular entities to monitor off-label use, dosing, and vulnerable populations.

  Example*:* For sotorasib, Amgen's DUS combined U.S. Symphony Health claims and Flatiron EHR to show 22% off-label use in non-G12C NSCLC within 6 months - triggering a regulatory safety review and updated SmPC wording [11].

- **Benefit confirmation (real-world response)**: How many patients taking the drug achieve clinically meaningful outcomes?

  Example: In support of pembrolizumab's landmark 2017 tumor-agnostic accelerated approval - the first tissue-agnostic FDA approval in oncology - the FDA accepted pooled data from five single-arm clinical trials enrolling 149 patients with MSI-H/dMMR solid tumors across 15 tumor types, demonstrating an objective response rate of 39.6% (95% CI 31.7–47.9%) with durable responses in 78% of responders at six months or more [12]. This precedent-setting approval was subsequently reinforced by real-world effectiveness studies confirming comparable clinical benefit in routine practice.

- **Comparative effectiveness**: Payers require head-to-head evidence in routine care.

  Example: A target trial emulation using electronic health records from a large US academic health system compared dupilumab, omalizumab, and mepolizumab in patients with moderate-to-severe asthma eligible for multiple biologics. Over 12 months of follow-up in 201 patients, dupilumab was associated with a lower rate of asthma-related exacerbations compared with omalizumab (adjusted incidence rate ratio [IRR] 0.36; 95% CI 0.12–1.09) and mepolizumab (IRR 0.28; 95% CI 0.09–0.84) - evidence that has informed biologic sequencing recommendations in severe asthma management [13].

### 14.1.4. Mature Product

This phase spans from third year post-launch to patent expiry. As generics/biosimilars approach, RWE shifts from demonstrating to sustaining value - often through adherence and subgroup evidence. The goal is to Defend pricing, expand indications, enable value-based contracts.

Evidence needs:

- **Adherence and persistence**: Critical for performance-based contracts.

  Example: A retrospective US claims study of 6,934 multiple sclerosis patients initiating oral disease-modifying therapies found teriflunomide and fingolimod demonstrated superior 12-month persistence (60%, 66%) and adherence versus dimethyl fumarate (44%, 40%) and diroximel fumarate (49%, 44%), allowing RWE to justify these products' clinical and economic value in a competitive market. [12].

- **Long-term safety and effectiveness**: This generally translates into 3+ year cohorts to detect delayed risks and benefits.

  Example: The CVD-REAL 3 study linked national registries across 11 countries (n = 900,000) to confirm SGLT2 inhibitors reduce heart failure hospitalizations by 39% over 3.2 years in average - extending findings beyond RCT follow-up and influencing ADA/EASD guidelines [15].

- **Subgroup value**: Real-world evidence in underrepresented populations justifies premium pricing.

  Example: The OSI-FACT-EP study confirmed osimertinib's effectiveness in elderly patients (75+ years) with advanced NSCLC. In this real-world setting, median PFS reached 19.1 months, mirroring the landmark FLAURA trial's 18.9 months. This RWE validates the product's value in "fragile" subgroups, supporting its standard-of-care position for mature market life-cycle management [16].

## 14.1.5. Post-Patent

Even after loss of exclusivity, RWE remains strategic - for biosimilars, repurposing, or policy. The goal is to differentiate, repurpose, and extend public health impact.

The evidence needs include:

- **Biosimilar uptake and switching**: DUS can be used to monitor real-world interchangeability.

  Example: The DANBIO registry study analyzed a Danish nationwide mandate switching 802 patients from originator infliximab to a biosimilar. This real-world DUS showed no significant changes in disease activity or 1-year retention rates (84.1%), providing critical RWE that supported large-scale biosimilar uptake and cost-saving switching policies globally [17].

- **Repurposing via RWE discovery**: Hypothesis generation followed by RCT confirmation.

  Example: Prior observational data suggested a potential anti-inflammatory benefit of colchicine in coronary artery disease, motivating the COLCOT (Colchicine Cardiovascular Outcomes Trial). This randomized trial of 4,745 patients with recent myocardial infarction confirmed a 23% relative reduction (HR 0.77; 95% CI 0.61–0.96; p=0.02) in the primary cardiovascular composite endpoint with low-dose colchicine 0.5 mg daily - evidence that underpinned FDA's 2023 approval of low-dose colchicine (Lodoco) for cardiovascular risk reduction in patients with established atherosclerotic disease [18].

- **Public health surveillance**: Long-term population impact.

  Example: A nested case-control study used Kaiser Permanente data to analyze rofecoxib after five years on the market. It identified a 3.7-fold increase in heart attack risk among high-dose users, contributing to the drug's 2004 withdrawal and the creation of the FDA's proactive Sentinel Initiative for public health surveillance. [19].

This lifecycle lens ensures RWE is neither over-engineered too early nor under-invested too late. A product's evidence plan should be as dynamic as its development path - iterative, responsive, and grounded in real-world learning. Integrated evidence generation planning (IEGP) aims to satisfy this goal.

## 14.2. Alignment of Evidence Needs, Study Designs and Data Sources

Before selecting designs, we must clarify what our stakeholders need to know. Critically, many of these needs cannot be addressed by randomized trials alone. For instance:

- **Natural history** for ultra-rare diseases often relies on registries or literature reviews - RCTs are infeasible.

- **Drug utilization** and treatment patterns happens by definition outside the realm of clinical trials.
- **Long-term safety** of chronic therapies often requires prospective cohort or active surveillance, as trial follow-up is limited.
- **Adherence and persistence** is purposefully measured in real-life.
- **Patient experience and equity** demand direct patient input (surveys, PROs), which RCTs systematically underrepresent.

Thus, RWE is not a "second-best" alternative in these cases - it is the only feasible and ethical way to answer many high-stakes questions. The challenge is to run the right study which can address the right need.

Clearly, the study design and the choice of data source shall be dictated by the research question. In practice, multiple solutions could be proposed for answering each evidence need. However, each stakeholder has their own preferences, justified by their ultimate goals. This is why understanding the subjacent goals behind the requests of regulators and payers is important in selecting the right study design and data sources. Table 14.1 provides a snapshot of typical study designs and data sources per evidence needs along with real-world examples.

## 14.3. Evidence Strategy Planning in Practice

In practice, **evidence strategy planning** is a multi-stakeholder exercise which is conducted and matured through iteration. Several actions are undertaken with the specific product or franchise in mind:

- **Stakeholder & Decision Context**: "Who needs the evidence? (Regulator / Payer / Clinician / Patient)"

**Table 14.1 Evidence Needs per Lifecyle Phase along with Typical Study Designs and Data Sources**

| Real-World Evidence Need | Lifecycle Phase(s) | Typical Study Design(s) | Typical Data Source(s) | Real-World Example |
|---|---|---|---|---|
| **Epidemiology** | Pre-/ Peri-Approval | Prospective or retrospective cohort | Disease registry, EHR, Claims | SOD1-ALS prevalence via Project MinE [4,5] |
| **Standard of care** | Pre-/ Peri-Approval | Cohort, Cross-sectional physician survey, Chart review | Physician survey, EHR, Claims | SoC mapping for sotorasib [6] |
| **Burden of illness** | Pre-/Peri-Approval | Retrospective cohort + PRO survey | Claims, Registry, Patient survey | ATTR amyloidosis burden for vutrisiran [7] |
| **Trial eligibility** | Pre-approval | Cross sectional | Claims, EHR | Checking eligible patients |
| **Budget Impact** | Peri-approval | Simulation | RCT, RWE, RWD | Lecanemab study [9] |
| **Measure of exposure** | Peri-Approval, Early Post-Approval | DUS, Claims trend analysis | Claims, EHR, Pharmacy records | Sotorasib DUS (off-label use) [11] |
| **Drug utilization** | Peri-/Early Post-Approval | Cohort (retrospective preferred), cross sectional | Claims, EHR, Registry | Sotorasib DUS [11] |
| **Safety evaluation** | Early Post-Approval, Mature Product | Prospective/retrospective PASS/PMS, Active surveillance | Registry, EHR, Sentinel, Darwin EU | CVD-REAL 3 Study for SGLT2 inhibitors [15] |
| **Effectiveness evaluation** | Early Post-Approval | Cohort with Target trial emulation | EHR, Registry, Claims | Dupilumab comparison study [13] |
| **Compliance/ adherence** | Mature Product | Sensor-enabled monitoring, Claims | Claims, PRO, Survey, Apps | Teriflunomide in MS [12] |

- **Core Evidence Need:** "What is the primary question? (e.g., long-term safety, comparative effectiveness, burden of illness)"
- **Top 2–3 Design Options**: listing 2–3 designs (e.g., for long-term safety: "Prospective PASS cohort", "Target trial emulation using linked claims and EHR", "Active surveillance")
- **Data Fitness Check**: "Do you have access to the data for this design?"
    - *Yes*: Proceed to study concept sheet development & pre-specification
    - *No*: Iterate (e.g., add PRO survey to claims study) or downgrade ambition (e.g., hypothesis-generating only)

The process is iterative and involves several rounds of discussions among stakeholders. Even after the finalization of evidence strategy plan, it is very likely to change. Indeed, the life of the product itself is subject to change due to unexpected uptake, introduction of competitors, or changes in the regulatory and reimbursement landscape.

The product evidence strategy plan shall therefore be *revised regularly* to reflect not only the changes of the product life cycle itself, but also the pitfalls of the current plan, and mitigate the risks. For example, if a decided and scheduled study fails to recruit, or a given data source becomes unavailable due to a new data privacy regulation, the product owner needs to find another way to address its evidence needs and fulfill its commitments. This is why in an evidence strategy plan, often times a risk evaluation and mitigation plan is also included.

### 14.3.1. A hypothetical example

To operationalize the principles outlined above - and to demonstrate how evidence strategy planning functions as a coherent, longitudinal roadmap - Table 14.2 presents a hypothetical real-world exemple: **semaglutide**, from early development through to its mature product phase and biosimilar horizon. We reconstruct here a hypothetical and simplified plan as if it was created earlier in the product life cycle. This single-product narrative illustrates how stakeholder needs evolve across the lifecycle, and how each need is addressed by a fit-for-purpose pairing of study design and data source - graded and justified in alignment with the evidence needs. The table includes practical considerations often overlooked in guidance documents - cost, timeline, and real-world feasibility. Rather than a collection of isolated studies, this is evidence strategy: iterative, anticipatory, and anchored in decision context.

## 14.4. Pitfalls and Mitigation Strategies

Even with a well-structured evidence strategy, execution risks can undermine credibility - not because of flawed statistics, but because of mismatches between intention and implementation. These pitfalls fall into four archetypes:

- **Temporal misalignment** (e.g., investing in long-term registries before confirming target validation),
- **Fitness overstatement** (e.g., claiming "real-world effectiveness" from a claims-only study lacking clinical endpoints),
- **Stakeholder misreading** (e.g., submitting a drug utilization study to a payer without linking exposure to outcomes or cost), and
- **Context blindness** (e.g., ignoring data latency in fast-evolving therapeutic areas like oncology or digital health).

Preventive mitigation of these pitfalls is paramount, as when they happen it is often too late to compensate for the lost time and investment. Critically, these are not merely methodological oversights - they reflect gaps in strategic coherence between the evidence need, the chosen design, and the decision context. Table 14.3 outlines common pitfalls with their real-world consequences, and pragmatic, fitness-preserving mitigation strategies - emphasizing that robust RWE begins not with analysis, but with alignment.

**Table 14.2 A Simplified Hypothetical Evidence Strategy Plan for Semaglutide**

| Phase | Stakeholder | Need | Design | Data Source | Rationale | Cost | Time | Example Study |
|---|---|---|---|---|---|---|---|---|
| **Pre-Approval** | Regulators (FDA/EMA), Pharma | Epidemio-logy & burden | Cohort, Survey | NHANES, GBD | Nationally representative (NHANES); global burden estimates (GBD) | $ | + | GBD Obesity Analysis |
| **Peri-Approval** | Payers (HAS), Pharma | Budget impact, SoC | Forecasting, Survey | SNDS, Physician Survey | SNDS: national coverage; survey: prescribing intent | $$ | ++ | Semaglutide Budget Impact Model |
| **Early Post-Approval** | Regulators (FDA) | Long-term safety | PMS/ PASS | Sentinel System | Active surveillance; pre-specified protocol | $$$ | +++ | GLP-1 RA CV Safety Study |
| | Payers (ICER) | Real-world effectiveness | Target trial emulation | Optum EHR/Claims | EHR: outcomes; claims: persistence/costs | $$ | ++ | Semaglutide effectiveness study |
| **Mature Product** | Payers (CMS) | Adherence–outcome link | Cohort + Sensor | Claims + Proteus | Claims: PDC; sensors: objective adherence | $$$ | +++ | Semaglutide Adherence-Outcomes Study |
| | Public Health | Equity of access | Federated cohort | SNDS + ZIP/ADI | SNDS: national; ADI: SDOH proxy | $ | + | Semaglutide Equity Analysis |
| **Post-Patent** | Regulators (EMA) | Biosimilar switching | Claims trend + Survey | German AOK + PRO | AOK: large cohort; PRO: symptom stability | $$ | ++ | GLP-1 Biosimilar Switching |

**Table 14.3 Example Pitfalls and Mitigation Strategies**

| Pitfall | Example | Mitigation |
|---|---|---|
| **Mismatched pairing** | Using social media (E) for long-term safety | Reserve for signal generation; confirm with EHR/registry |
| **Ignoring stakeholder criteria** | Submitting DUS to NICE without cost-effectiveness linkage | Co-develop protocol early via Scientific Advice (FDA/EMA/NICE) |
| **Single-source overreliance** | EHR-only study missing OTC drug use | Link EHR + pharmacy claims + patient-reported meds |
| **Latency blindness** | Using 2022 claims for 2024 SoC (post-pandemic shifts) | Supplement with rapid-cycle survey (e.g., 4-week physician pulse) |

## 14.5. Global Variation in Design Acceptance

The "fitness" of a study design-data source pairing is not absolute - it is shaped by regional regulatory philosophies, health system infrastructure, and historical precedent. A design considered as acceptable in one jurisdiction may be possible but high risk or even considered unacceptable in another, not due to methodological flaws, but because of differing expectations around prospectivity, data provenance, or stakeholder engagement.

For instance, EMA's emphasis on prospective data generation for post-authorisation efficacy studies (PAES) elevates registry-based cohorts, while retrospective EHR analyses - though accepted by FDA for label expansions - often require supplemental validation to meet EU standards. A frequent confusion is about external control arms: FDA expects them when the conditions of a randomized double-arm trial are not met, whereas EMA considers that in those cases the single arm trial shall be self-sufficient. Similarly, HAS's requirement for mixed-methods evidence in high-budget impact assessments renders claims-only studies insufficient, whereas PMDA may accept cross-sectional surveys where EHR interoperability remains limited. This variation is not arbitrary: it reflects deliberate trade-offs between rigour, timeliness, and feasibility - and must be anticipated in any global evidence strategy. Table 14.4

provides a few typical examples. An interesting observation is that these positions can evolve.

**Table 14.4 Variation in Design Acceptance**

| Region | Key Distinction | Impact on Fitness |
|---|---|---|
| **EU (EMA)** | High bar for *prospective* data in PAES/PASS; registries privileged, considers external control arms as nice, but not necessary | Retrospective EHR study is less preferred in comparative effectiveness (unless supplemented with prospective validation) |
| **U.S. (FDA)** | Accepts well-conducted retrospective RWE for label expansions if protocol pre-specified, external control arms are part of its framework | Target trial emulation with EHR is preferred |
| **France (HAS)** | Requires *mixed methods* for PAMs: quantitative (SNDS) + qualitative (PRO/survey) | Claims-only study is less preferred for high-impact decisions |
| **Japan (PMDA)** | Prioritizes longitudinal national databases (NDB, MHW) for aging populations | Cross-sectional survey is less preferred unless part of iterative learning system |
| **LMICs (WHO)** | Feasibility-driven: mobile surveys, facility logs often accepted | EHR-based cohort is less accepted if system coverage <20% |

## 14.5.1. The Need for a Purpose-Driven and Widely Accepted Evidence Alignment

Traditional hierarchies of evidence - ranking study designs by methodological form rather than functional fit - have long shaped how we evaluate research. Yet in real-world decision-making, fitness for purpose consistently outweighs design taxonomy. A retrospective cohort may provide more credible evidence of long-term safety than a short-term pragmatic trial; a well-conducted literature review may better define natural history for an ultra-rare disease than a newly launched registry with slow accrual.

The challenge is not merely conceptual: it is operational. Stakeholders routinely face trade-offs between scientific rigor, timeliness, cost, and feasibility. Yet few practical tools exist to guide these choices, particularly ones that integrate stakeholder context, evidence need, design options, data source suitability, and resource implications into a single, transparent framework.

There is a clear need - and growing momentum - for **a dynamic, evidence-based alignment matrix**: one that moves beyond static hierarchies to support proportional study selection. Such a matrix would not dictate answers, but illuminate pathways - helping teams ask: "Is this the simplest credible approach to answer this question, for this decision, at this time?"

In 2023 the author gathered a group of expert from different horizons to develop such a matrix. The outcome, the ALIGN matrix will be published soon.

## 14.6. Integrated Evidence Generation (IEG)

### 14.6.1. Strategic Architecture and Core Principles

Integrated evidence generation (IEG) moves beyond parallel study execution to create a unified evidence architecture that prospectively aligns clinical trials, real-world data, health economics, patient-reported outcomes, and biomarker insights around shared decision contexts. Rather than treating RWE as a post-hoc supplement or a siloed compliance exercise, IEG positions it as a continuous calibration layer that stress-tests trial assumptions, contextualizes efficacy within routine practice, and quantifies multidimensional value.

At its core, IEG is governed by three interlocking principles.

- First, prospective convergence ensures that trial protocols, observational studies, and economic models are co-developed with harmonized endpoints, shared data dictionaries, and aligned causal assumptions.
- Second, cross-validation leverages the complementary strengths of each stream: randomized trials establish internal validity and dose-response relationships, real-world studies

confirm external validity and long-term performance, health economic models translate clinical outcomes into budget impact, and patient-centered data captures dimensions of value that traditional endpoints miss.

- Third, adaptive continuity guarantees that the evidence portfolio remains responsive to emerging safety signals, competitive shifts, and evolving payer expectations without compromising methodological integrity or governance standards. This principled architecture transforms fragmented data points into a coherent decision framework, ensuring that every study answers a specific piece of a larger stakeholder puzzle.

### 14.6.2. Operational Execution and Lifecycle Integration

Operationalizing IEG requires deliberate cross-functional governance and shared technical infrastructure. Evidence teams spanning clinical development, pharmacoepidemiology, market access, medical affairs, and data science must establish a master evidence protocol that defines priority questions, assigns complementary study roles, and pre-specifies integration rules. Shared data infrastructure becomes critical: interoperable EHR-claims-linkage pipelines, standardized ontologies, and FAIR-compliant repositories enable seamless evidence synthesis while reducing redundant data collection and minimizing bias propagation.

When regulatory submissions, HTA dossiers, and clinical guidelines draw from the same integrated evidence base, the risk of contradictory conclusions diminishes and stakeholder trust accelerates.

Throughout the product lifecycle, IEG functions as a continuous learning loop rather than a static deliverable.

- **Pre-approval**, it aligns target validation with burden-of-illness metrics and standard-of-care mapping.
- **Peri-approval**, it synchronizes budget impact forecasts with early access program data and risk mitigation workflows.

- **Post-approval**, it links long-term safety surveillance with adherence patterns, comparative effectiveness, and value-based contracting thresholds.

By anchoring every evidence activity to a unified decision architecture, sponsors transform isolated studies into strategic assets. IEG is no longer an academic ideal; it is the foundational operating system for sustainable development, regulatory success, and equitable patient access in an era where therapeutic value is defined by real-world performance.

## 14.7. Conclusion

Evidence is not neutral - it is shaped by the lens of the questioner. A regulator evaluating benefit–risk, a payer assessing value, a clinician optimizing care, and a patient prioritizing autonomy all need different kinds of evidence.

This chapter provided a structured way to align RWE generation with that diversity - not through rigid prescription, but through purpose-driven matching:

*Evidence need → Study design → Data source → Fitness validation.*

By anchoring study selection in stakeholder decision contexts, we move from producing RWE to producing usable RWE - evidence that informs, persuades, and ultimately improves health outcomes.

### References

1. U.S. Food and Drug Administration. Considerations for the Use of Real-World Data and Real-World Evidence to Support Regulatory Decision-Making for Drug and Biological Products. Guidance for Industry. Silver Spring (MD): FDA; 2023.

2. EMA. Reflection paper on use of real-world data in non-interventional studies to generate real-world evidence. EMA/519347/2023. Amsterdam: European Medicines Agency; 2024.

3. ISPOR. HTA-Ready Value Dossiers: A Global Roadmap. 2023.

4. Opie-Martin S, Iacoangeli A, Topp SD, et al. The SOD1-mediated ALS phenotype shows a decoupling between age of symptom onset and disease duration. Nat Commun. 2022 Nov 12;13:6901.

5. Miller TM, Cudkowicz ME, Genge A, et al. Trial of Antisense Oligonucleotide Tofersen for SOD1 ALS. N Engl J Med. 2022;387(12):1099–1110.

6. Gray JE, Hsu H, Younan D, et al. Real-world outcomes in patients with KRAS G12C-mutated advanced non-small cell lung cancer treated with docetaxel in second-line or beyond. Lung Cancer. 2023;181:107260.

7. Ruberg FL, Grogan M, Hanna M, et al. Transthyretin amyloid cardiomyopathy: JACC state-of-the-art review. J Am Coll Cardiol. 2019;73(22):2872–2891.

8. Murthy VH, Krumholz HM, Gross CP. Participation in cancer clinical trials: race-, sex-, and age-based disparities. JAMA. 2004;291(22):2720–2726.

9. van Dyck CH, Swanson CJ, Aisen P, et al. Lecanemab in Early Alzheimer's Disease. N Engl J Med. 2023;388(1):9–21.

10. Schuster SJ, Bishop MR, Tam CS, et al. Tisagenlecleucel in Adult Relapsed or Refractory Diffuse Large B-Cell Lymphoma. N Engl J Med. 2019;380(1):45–56.

11. FDA. Sotorasib Post-Marketing Requirement: Drug Utilization Study (NCT05244540). Silver Spring (MD): U.S. Food and Drug Administration; 2023.

12. Marcus L, Lemery SJ, Keegan P, Pazdur R. FDA Approval Summary: Pembrolizumab for the Treatment of Microsatellite Instability-High Solid Tumors. Clin Cancer Res. 2019;25(13):3753–3758.

13. Akenroye AT, Segal JB, Zhou G, et al. Comparative effectiveness of omalizumab, mepolizumab, and dupilumab in asthma: a target trial emulation. J Allergy Clin Immunol. 2023;151(5):1269–1276.

14. Araujo L, Geertsen SS, Amedume A, et al. Persistence, adherence, and switching to higher-cost therapy in patients with multiple

sclerosis initiating oral disease-modifying therapies: a retrospective real-world study. Neurol Ther. 2022;11(4):1735-1748.

15. Wilding JP, Batterham RL, Calanna S, et al. Once-Weekly Semaglutide in Adults with Overweight or Obesity. N Engl J Med. 2021;384(11):989–1002.

16. Nakao A, Fukui T, Uchida N, et al. Osimertinib as first-line treatment for elderly patients with advanced EGFR mutation-positive non-small cell lung cancer in a real-world setting (OSI-FACT-EP). Thorac Cancer. 2022;13(21):3031-3038.

17. Glintborg B, Sørensen IJ, Loft AG, Lindegaard H, Linauskas A, Hendricks O, et al. A nationwide non-medical switch from originator infliximab to biosimilar CT-P13 in 802 patients with inflammatory arthritis: 1-year clinical outcomes from the DANBIO registry. *Annals of the Rheumatic Diseases*. 2017 Aug;76(8):1426-1431.

18. Tardif JC, Kouz S, Waters DD, et al. Efficacy and Safety of Low-Dose Colchicine after Myocardial Infarction. N Engl J Med. 2019;381(26):2497–2505.

19. Graham DJ, Campen D, Hui R, et al. Risk of acute myocardial infarction and sudden cardiac death in patients treated with cyclo-oxygenase 2 selective and non-selective non-steroidal anti-inflammatory drugs: nested case-control study. *The Lancet*. 2005 Feb 5;365(9458):475-481.

# Chapter 15. Real-World Evidence and Digital Health

The convergence of digital health technologies and real-world evidence (RWE) is accelerating the generation of high-frequency, patient-centric data streams that were previously inaccessible in traditional clinical research. Unlike administrative databases or retrospective electronic health record (EHR) analyses, digital health tools enable continuous, longitudinal observation of health states, behaviors, and physiological parameters - often in near real time.

This chapter explores how three core categories - wearables, remote monitoring systems, and digital biomarkers - are reshaping RWE collection, validation, and application. WhilePart I: Chapter 2. Chapter 2. introduced the types of real-world data (RWD), and Chapter 13. discussed how industry leverages RWE for safety and effectiveness, here the emphasis is on how digital health innovations are expanding the scope, granularity, and timeliness of RWE - particularly for dynamic endpoints and patient-reported outcomes.

## 15.1. Wearables

Wearable devices - such as smartwatches, fitness trackers, and medical-grade sensors - capture objective, high-resolution data on activity, heart rate, sleep patterns, oxygen saturation, and, increasingly, electrocardiography (ECG) and glucose trends. Their appeal in RWE lies not only in the volume of data but in the ability to monitor patients in naturalistic settings over extended periods without clinician intervention.

The evidentiary value of wearable data hinges on sensor reliability, algorithmic validation, and contextual interpretation. For example, the Apple Heart Study, a large prospective virtual trial, recruited over 419,297 participants via the Apple Watch to detect irregular pulse rhythms suggestive of atrial fibrillation. Among those who received notification of irregular pulse, 34% had atrial fibrillation on subsequent ECG patch readings among whom, 84% were ultimately concordant with atrial fibrillation [1]. While the study confirmed feasibility at scale – unprecedented in classic prospective study - it also revealed challenges in specificity and the need for confirmatory diagnostics - illustrating that raw sensor output alone rarely suffices as RWE; it must be embedded in a robust analytical framework.

Regulatory agencies have begun formalizing expectations. In 2023, the FDA issued Digital Health Technologies for Remote Data Acquisition in Clinical Investigations, providing recommendations on data provenance, metadata standards (e.g., timestamps, device ID), and algorithm transparency [2]. In 2025, the FDA supplemented this with guidance on the use of Artificial Intelligence (AI) and Machine Learning (ML) in medical device software, emphasizing the need for Predetermined Change Control Plans (PCCPs) to manage algorithmic drift in real-world settings [3].

Key considerations in using wearables for RWE include:

- **Device heterogeneity:** Consumer wearables vary widely in sampling frequency and algorithmic assumptions. Harmonization (e.g., via ISO/IEEE 11073 standards []) remains incomplete.

- **Data continuity bias:** Users may discontinue wearing devices, leading to missingness that correlates with health status (e.g., fatigue, worsening symptoms).
- **Contextual interpretation:** A step count alone is insufficient without covariates (e.g., disease severity, mobility aids). Linking wearable data to EHRs or patient-reported outcomes enhances interpretability.

## 15.2. Remote Monitoring

Remote monitoring extends beyond self-administered wearables to clinician-initiated, often condition-specific systems deployed in home or ambulatory settings. Typical modalities include connected blood pressure cuffs, weight scales for heart failure management, continuous glucose monitors (CGMs), respiratory monitors, and implantable telemetry (e.g., cardiac implantable electronic devices, CIEDs).

Remote monitoring data are uniquely valuable for capturing dynamic trajectories and early warning signals. For instance, a retrospective evaluation of a real-world U.S., connected cardiac care program (CCCP), the program involving daily telemonitoring of symptoms and vital signs demonstrated a 19% reduction in 30-day readmissions (HR)=0.52, 95% CI 0.31-0.86, *P*=.01) [4]. In the EU, the Telemedical Interventional Management in Heart Failure II (TIM-HF2) trial showed that structured telemonitoring improved outcomes and enabled earlier diuretic adjustments - evidence later cited in NICE guidance on the remote management of heart failure [5,6].

However, remote monitoring RWE demands rigorous attention to data governance. The International Council for Harmonisation (ICH) E6(R3) guideline (2025) introduces explicit guidance on source data verification for decentralized data streams, recommending that sponsors define trusted data streams - i.e., systems where data integrity, audit trails, and calibration are pre-validated [7].

Challenges specific to remote monitoring RWE include:

- **Calibration drift:** Sensor accuracy may degrade over time, especially in non-medical-grade devices; periodic recalibration or cross-validation with clinic measurements is essential.
- **Alert fatigue:** Over-sensitive algorithms can overwhelm care teams, leading to desensitization and missed critical events.
- **Equity of access:** Socioeconomic disparities in broadband, device ownership, and digital literacy can skew samples toward healthier, wealthier populations - a bias that must be quantified and mitigated (e.g., via inverse probability weighting or targeted recruitment).

### 15.2.1. Remote Monitoring RWE Protocol Checklist

To ensure methodological rigor, sponsors and investigators should verify the following items before initiating a remote monitoring RWE study.

- Define primary and secondary digital endpoints a priori
- Document device make, model, firmware version, and sampling frequency
- Establish data transmission latency thresholds (e.g., <2 hours for critical alerts)
- Specify data cleaning rules (e.g., outlier removal based on physiological plausibility)
- Pre-register data analysis plan in a public repository (e.g., OSF or protocol publication in ARWDE)

## 15.3. Digital Biomarkers

Digital biomarkers are objective, quantifiable physiological and behavioral measures collected and analyzed via digital devices, intended to serve as indicators of normal biological processes, pathogenic processes, or responses to an intervention [8]. Unlike traditional laboratory biomarkers, digital biomarkers often reflect functional status - e.g., gait speed derived from smartphone accelerometry in multiple sclerosis, or speech prosody changes detected by voice analysis in early Parkinson's disease.

The FDA has formalized a framework for utilizing Digital Health Technologies (DHTs) in drug development, often leveraging the Biomarker Qualification Program (BQP) for digital measures. Landmark examples include:

- **mPower Parkinson's** study pioneered the use of smartphone-based motor tasks to track disease severity, the FDA has issued formal Letters of Support for other digital measures, such as wearable-derived physical activity metrics in clinical trials [9].
- **Pear Therapeutics' reSET**, was the first FDA-authorized prescription digital therapeutic (PDT), which demonstrated significantly improved abstinence and treatment retention in a pivotal trial [10]. However, Pear's 2023 bankruptcy highlighted a persistent "reimbursement gap," illustrating that regulatory clearance and real-world evidence (RWE) do not automatically guarantee payer coverage.

In Europe, the Innovative Health Initiative (IHI) **RADAR-CNS** project developed and validated digital biomarkers for depression and epilepsy using multimodal smartphone and wearable data, culminating in an open-access analytical toolkit adopted by academic and industry partners [11,12].

Methodological pillars for credible digital biomarker RWE include:

- **Analytical validation:** Demonstrating that the digital signal accurately reflects the intended physiological parameter (e.g., algorithmic sensitivity/specificity against gold-standard measurements).
- **Clinical validation:** Establishing that the digital biomarker correlates with clinical outcomes or predicts disease progression/response.

- **Contextual validation:** Showing performance consistency across intended use settings (e.g., varying lighting, ambient noise, patient positioning).

A common pitfall is overfitting during algorithm development - where models perform exceptionally well in training datasets but fail in external validation. Transparent reporting via the **DECIDE-AI** framework (part of the family of AI reporting standards alongside **SPIRIT-AI** and **CONSORT-AI**) helps mitigate this risk by requiring detailed documentation of data origins, model stability, and human-AI interaction in early clinical phases. [13].

## 15.4. Integration with Existing RWE Infrastructure

Digital health-derived RWE rarely stands alone. To generate actionable insights, it must be integrated with traditional RWD sources - e.g., linking CGM glucose excursions to pharmacy claims for insulin use, or fusing wearable activity data with hospitalization records to model decompensation risk. Chapter 2. outlined data linkage basics; here we focus on operational and semantic interoperability challenges unique to digital streams.

Key standards facilitating integration include:

- **Fast Healthcare Interoperability Resources (FHIR)**: The HL7 FHIR Digital Health Devices (DHD) implementation guide (2023) defines resources for device metadata, observations, and alerts [14].
- **OMOP Common Data Model (CDM)**: The OHDSI community released updated Sensor Measurement standards to better accommodate high-frequency time-series data from consumer wearables [15].
- **ISO/TS 82304-2**: Specifies health and wellness apps' quality and safety requirements, aiding cross-study comparability [16].

A notable global example is the **All of Us Research Program**, which combines EHRs, genomics, and Fitbit wearables for participants, demonstrating scalable linkage architecture and participant-controlled data sharing [17]. It's worth noting that while the program has over 873,000 total participants today, the wearable segment is smaller because it requires a separate "Bring Your Own Device" (BYOD) authorization or participation in a specific device-distribution sub-study.

In Japan, the **Medical Information Database (MID-NET)** has been subsumed into the Nationwide Medical Information Platform. This cloud-based infrastructure now integrates electronic health records (EHRs) with high-frequency data from national telehealth and remote monitoring pilots, significantly expanding the PMDA's capacity for real-world pharmacoepidemiologic studies [18].

Nonetheless, integration introduces new bias vectors:

- **Temporal misalignment**: e.g., EHR lab draws at clinic visits vs. continuous CGM,
- **Scale mismatch**: claims coded in ICD-10 vs. second-by-second sensor logs,
- **Privacy–utility trade-offs**: e.g., aggregation thresholds that obscure individual trajectories.

Chapter 7. bias mitigation strategies - such as time-varying propensity scores and marginal structural models - are increasingly adapted for these hybrid data environments.

## 15.5. Ethical, Legal, and Regulatory Considerations

Digital health RWE raises distinctive ethical concerns, notably around informed consent scope, data sovereignty, and algorithmic transparency. The EU's General Data Protection Regulation (GDPR) Article 22 restricts fully automated decision-making affecting individuals, which constrains how digital biomarker alerts can trigger clinical actions without human oversight [19]. In contrast, the U.S. 21st Century Cures

Act promotes interoperability but delegates granular consent management to institutional review boards (IRBs), leading to heterogeneity in practice [20].

The FDA's **Digital Health Center of Excellence (DHCoE)** issued its landmark guidance regarding Predetermined Change Control Plans (PCCPs) for AI-enabled software. This framework provides a formal pathway for manufacturers to pre-specify and gain authorization for future algorithmic updates based on real-world data, ensuring that RWE-driven improvements do not require a new marketing submission for every iteration [21].

Meanwhile, the UK's MHRA concluded its initial "AI Airlock" regulatory sandbox pilot in 2025. The results provided a blueprint for managing "hallucinations" in Large Language Models (LLMs) used in clinical settings [22].

A recurring tension lies between data minimization (collect only what is necessary) and data richness (collect broadly for future discovery). Strategies such as **dynamic consent platforms** - where participants can adjust sharing permissions over time - and **federated learning** (model training without raw data leaving local sites) are gaining traction as pragmatic compromises.

## 15.6. Conclusion

Digital health technologies are transforming RWE from episodic, retrospectively assembled snapshots into continuous, prospective, and patient-centered evidence streams. Wearables provide scalable activity and physiological metrics, remote monitoring delivers condition-specific, high-fidelity data for chronic disease management, and digital biomarkers offer novel, functional endpoints that complement traditional clinical measures. Yet, the promise of digital RWE is matched by methodological, regulatory, and ethical complexities: sensor validation, algorithmic bias, data integration, and consent governance must be addressed systematically.

As these technologies mature, their role in regulatory submissions, health technology assessment, and clinical decision support will expand - especially for endpoints that are impractical to capture in RCTs, such as real-world adherence, functional mobility, or symptom burden trajectories. Future editions of this book will likely see digital health not as a distinct chapter, but as the **substrate** upon which much of RWE is built. For now, practitioners must balance innovation with rigor, ensuring that digital RWE meets the same standards of credibility, transparency, and patient relevance as evidence derived from more established sources.

## References

1. Perez MV, Mahaffey KW, Hedlin H, et al. Large-scale assessment of a smartwatch to identify atrial fibrillation. N Engl J Med. 2019;381(20):1909–1917.

2. U.S. Food and Drug Administration. Digital Health Technologies for Remote Data Acquisition in Clinical Investigations: Guidance for Industry, Investigators, and Other Stakeholders. Silver Spring, MD: FDA; 2023.

3. U.S. Food and Drug Administration. Marketing Submission Recommendations for a Predetermined Change Control Plan for Artificial Intelligence-Enabled Device Software Functions. Silver Spring, MD: FDA; 2025.

4. Agboola S, Jethwani K, Khateeb K, Moore S, Kvedar J. Heart failure remote monitoring: evidence from the retrospective evaluation of a real-world remote monitoring program. JMIR Mhealth Uhealth. 2015;3(2):e54.

4. Koehler K, Koehler S, Deckwart O, et al. Efficacy of telemedical interventional management in patients with heart failure (TIM-HF2): a randomised, controlled, parallel-group, unmasked trial. *Lancet.* 2018;392(10152):1047-57.

6. National Institute for Health and Care Excellence. (2020). myCOPD for self-management of chronic obstructive pulmonary disease. Medtech innovation briefing [MIB214]. https://www.nice.org.uk/advice/mib214

7. International Council for Harmonisation. Guideline for Good Clinical Practice E6(R3). Step 4 version. Geneva: ICH; 2025.

8. Babrak LM, Menetski J, Rebhan M, et al. Traditional and digital biomarkers: two worlds apart? Digit Biomark. 2019;3(2):92-102.

9. Bot BM, Suve C, Neto EC, et al. The mPower study, Parkinson disease mobile data collected using ResearchKit. Sci Data. 2016;3:160011. doi: 10.1038/sdata.2016.11.

10. Campbell AN, Nunes EV, Matthews AG et al. Internet-delivered treatment for substance abuse: a multi-site randomized controlled trial. Am J Psychiatry. 2014;171(6):683-90. doi: 10.1176/appi.ajp.2014.13081055.

11. Matcham F, Barattieri di San Pietro C, Bulgari V, et al. Remote assessment of disease and relapse in central nervous system disorders: mobile health studies in depression, multiple sclerosis, and epilepsy. Health Informatics J. 2019;25(4):1170-1182.

12. Innovative Health Initiative. RADAR-CNS: Remote assessment of disease and relapse in central nervous system disorders. Brussels: IHI; 2022 [cited 2026 May 4]. Available from: https://www.ihi.europa.eu/projects-results/project-factsheets/radar-cns

13. Vasey B, Nagendran M, Campbell B, et al. Reporting guideline for the early-stage clinical evaluation of decision support systems driven by artificial intelligence: DECIDE-AI. Nat Med. 2022;28(5):924-933. doi:10.1038/s41591-022-01772-9.

14. HL7 International. HL7 FHIR Implementation Guide: Digital Health Devices (DHD), Release 1. Ann Arbor (MI): HL7 International; 2023.

15. Observational Health Data Sciences and Informatics (OHDSI). OMOP Common Data Model v5.4: Sensor Table [Internet]. OHDSI; 2023.

16. International Organization for Standardization. ISO/TS 82304-2:2022 Health and wellness apps - Part 2: Quality and reliability. Geneva: ISO; 2022.

17. All of Us Research Program Investigators, Denny JC, Rutter JL, et al. The "All of Us" Research Program. N Engl J Med. 2019 Aug 15;381(7):668-676. doi: 10.1056/NEJMsr1809937.

18. Pharmaceuticals and Medical Devices Agency (PMDA). Promotion of Medical DX and the Nationwide Medical Information Platform: Integration of Real-World Data. Tokyo: MHLW/PMDA; 2025.

19. Regulation (EU) 2016/679 of the European Parliament and of the Council of 27 April 2016 on the protection of natural persons with regard to the processing of personal data and on the free movement of such data, and repealing Directive 95/46/EC (General Data Protection Regulation). Official Journal of the European Union. 2016 May 4;L119:1-88.

20. 21st Century Cures Act, Pub. L. No. 114-255, 130 Stat. 1033 (2016 Dec 13).

21. U.S. Food and Drug Administration. Marketing Submission Recommendations for a Predetermined Change Control Plan for Artificial Intelligence-Enabled Device Software Functions: Guidance for Industry and Food and Drug Administration Staff. Silver Spring (MD): FDA; 2024 Dec 4 (revised 2025 Aug 18). Docket No. FDA-2022-D-2628.

22. Medicines and Healthcare products Regulatory Agency. AI Airlock Sandbox Pilot Programme Report and Phase 2 Launch. London: MHRA; 2025.

# Chapter 16. The Future of Real-World Evidence

The field of real-world evidence (RWE) has evolved from a niche supplement to randomized controlled trials (RCTs) into a foundational pillar of modern healthcare evidence generation. As regulatory acceptance grows and data ecosystems become increasingly sophisticated, the trajectory of RWE points toward deeper integration with advanced analytics, hybrid trial methodologies, and dynamic, learning health systems.

This chapter explores four interrelated frontiers that are poised to define the next decade of RWE:

- **Artificial Intelligence (AI)** and its transformative role;
- **Real-World Trials (RWT)**, particularly pragmatic and hybrid designs, that intentionally leverage routine clinical data infrastructure;
- **Continuous Evidence Ecosystems (CEEs)** though which evidence is generated and acted upon in near real time; and

- **RWD&E Discipline** as a standalone professional domain, thanks to the evolution of science, practice and infrastructure.

While each of these trends is technically distinct, their convergence signals a fundamental shift: from episodic evidence generation to embedded, continuous evidence synthesis as a routine component of care delivery.

## 16.1. Artificial Intelligence and RWE

Artificial intelligence, broadly encompassing machine learning (ML), natural language processing (NLP), and large language models (LLMs), offers both promise and complexity for RWE. Early applications focused on automating labor-intensive tasks - such as identifying patient cohorts from electronic health records (EHRs) or extracting structured variables from unstructured clinical notes, or predictive analytics [1].

However, the frontier now lies in augmenting scientific reasoning. Examples include conducting literature reviews, generating study documents, hypotheses (from longitudinal patient trajectories), correcting for unmeasured confounding through causal ML, and predicting treatment effect heterogeneity at the individual level. Table 16.1 presents some examples of AI-enabled RWE applications.

A key enabler has been the development of **foundation models** tailored to biomedical data. For instance, models such as Med-PaLM and ClinicalBERT have shown strong performance in clinical concept extraction and temporal reasoning when fine-tuned on real-world datasets [2].

In Europe, the **EHDS (European Health Data Space)** initiative explicitly identifies AI-ready health datasets as a strategic asset, with pilot projects testing ML-driven safety signal detection in distributed EHR networks across Germany, France, and the Netherlands [3].

**Table 16.1 Selected AI-enabled RWE Applications**

| Domain | Example | Data Source | Key Innovation | Region |
|---|---|---|---|---|
| **Safety surveillance** | Unsupervised clustering of longitudinal clinical measurements for adverse event pattern discovery | Multi-institutional EHRs (Cleveland Clinic system) | Integration of unsupervised learning with temporal clustering | United States [4] |
| **Effectiveness heterogeneity** | Heterogeneous cardiovascular effects of SGLT2 inhibitors in type 2 diabetes using causal forest with target trial emulation | Japanese administrative claims and registry data | Causal forest method with counterfactual risk adjustment to estimate individualized treatment effects | Japan [5] |
| **Operational efficiency** | Dynamic resource allocation for sepsis care using reinforcement learning on ICU monitoring streams | MIMIC-IV + hospital administrative data | Online policy optimization with bias-corrected reward estimation | Worldwide (open-source dataset) [6] |
| **RWE education / operational efficiency** | Live development of study concept sheet, protocol, statistical analysis plan, statistical codes, table shells, report, and its appraisal | Synthetic patient data + a body of knowledge on RWD/E | Integration of AI into the design and conduct of RWE study workflow with human review rounds in between steps | EvidenceAi™ Suite evidencemastery.com |
| **Public health** | ARGONet machine learning ensemble forecasts influenza across France regions | EHR, Web searches, climatic data | Multi-layered AI integration: nowcasting (real-time) & forecasting (future) | France [7] |

Nevertheless, AI introduces novel methodological challenges. Unlike classical regression models, many ML algorithms are "black boxes," raising concerns about interpretability, reproducibility, and transportability across health systems [8]. The FDA's AI/ML Software as a Medical Device (SaMD) Action Plan acknowledges this and calls for "good machine learning practice" (GMLP), including external validation on diverse populations and transparent model documentation [9].

In Europe, a notable example is the HealthData@EU pilot project with a deep learning algorithm to identify potential drug-induced liver injury signals in EHR data; the project required not only algorithmic validation but also clinician-in-the-loop adjudication to ensure clinical plausibility [10].

To advance responsibly, several consensus frameworks are emerging to standardize the reporting and stewardship of healthcare artificial intelligence. The TRIPOD+AI statement - which builds a 27-item checklist upon the foundational TRIPOD checklist - provides expanded guidance for the transparent reporting of AI-augmented studies using prediction models, specifically emphasizing data provenance, preprocessing pipelines, and model performance metrics across diverse subgroups [11]. Similarly, the FUTURE-AI framework - an international consensus guideline - incorporates principles of fairness and traceability, advocating for the systematic use of model cards and dataset sheets to ensure healthcare AI systems are transparent and facilitate replication [12].

## 16.2. From Pragmatism to Embedded, Continuous Evidence

While AI augments analysis, **real-world trials (RWTs)** reshape how interventions are evaluated. The term encompasses pragmatic randomized trials (PCTs), registry-based trials, and hybrid designs that randomize patients within routine clinical workflows while relying on existing data infrastructure for follow-up.

A defining characteristic is the minimization of research overhead. Eligibility criteria are broad, consent processes are streamlined (often using tiered or opt-out models where ethically and legally permissible), and outcome ascertainment leverages EHRs, claims, or patient-reported outcome (PRO) platforms rather than dedicated research visits. This increases external validity and scalability - but also demands rigorous attention to data completeness and protocol adherence in uncontrolled settings.

The ADAPTABLE trial in the United States exemplifies this **hybrid trial** approach [13]. Sponsored by PCORI, it randomized over 15,000 patients with established cardiovascular disease to aspirin 81 mg vs 325 mg using a decentralized, site-minimal model: recruitment occurred via mail and phone, consent was electronic, and outcomes (MI, stroke, death, bleeding) were ascertained through Medicare claims, commercial claims, and the Social Security Death Index. The trial completed enrollment in 22 months (vs projected 36) and demonstrated feasible large-scale pragmatic execution - though challenges persisted in outcome verification, leading to subsequent investment in NLP for bleeding event adjudication.

In Europe, the EU-PEARL project has pioneered master protocols for **Integrated Research Platforms (IRPs)**, developing a data infrastructure that allows patient data to be pulled directly from electronic health records (EHRs) and national registries for trial feasibility and pre-screening [14]. While EU-PEARL established these methodologies across Major Depressive Disorder, Tuberculosis, NASH, and Neurofibromatosis, its framework is designed to be disease-agnostic. For instance, in the Alzheimer's disease domain, the closely related ROADMAP project demonstrated the power of this approach by integrating real-world data from the Swedish Dementia Registry, the UK's NIHR Clinical Research Network, and Germany's AOK claims database to support evidence-generation for adaptive trials [15].

A newer evolution is the **embedded pragmatic clinical trial (ePCT)**, where the intervention is delivered as part of routine care, and randomization is triggered by clinical decision support (CDS) alerts. The Diuretic Comparison Project (DCP) trial in the US Department of Veterans Affairs tested two diuretics, namely Hydrochlorothiazide (HCTZ) and chlorthalidone (CTD) embedding allocation logic into the CDS workflow of the VA's EHR [16].

The study was conducted by a centralized research team with site procedures embedded in the electronic health record and all data collected through administrative claims data, with no study related visits for participants.

Figure 16.1 shows its conceptual diagram. This "research as care" model eliminates separate research infrastructure and enables rapid iteration - though it requires close collaboration between clinicians, informaticians, and institutional review boards.

## 16.3. Toward Learning Health Systems

The most ambitious vision for RWE's future is the **continuous evidence ecosystem** - a system in which data collection, analysis, and decision support operate in tight feedback loops, enabling evidence to be refreshed as care evolves. Unlike traditional studies with fixed start/end dates, continuous ecosystems treat evidence generation as an operational function, akin to laboratory testing or radiology reporting.

The foundational architecture consists of three pillars:

1. **Interoperable data fabrics** linking EHRs, claims, registries, and patient-generated data via standardized APIs (e.g., FHIR);
2. **Analytic pipelines** that run validated algorithms at scheduled intervals or in response to triggers (e.g., new drug approval, outbreak alert);
3. **Evidence delivery mechanisms** such as dynamic clinical guidelines, risk-stratified dashboards, or CDS updates informed by the latest RWE.

A pioneering example is the UK's OpenSAFELY platform [17]. Built on a privacy preserving model where code is sent to data (not vice versa), it processes over 58 million primary care records in near real time. During the pandemic, OpenSAFELY supported >30 rapid studies on vaccine effectiveness and drug safety, with protocols pre-registered and code fully open.

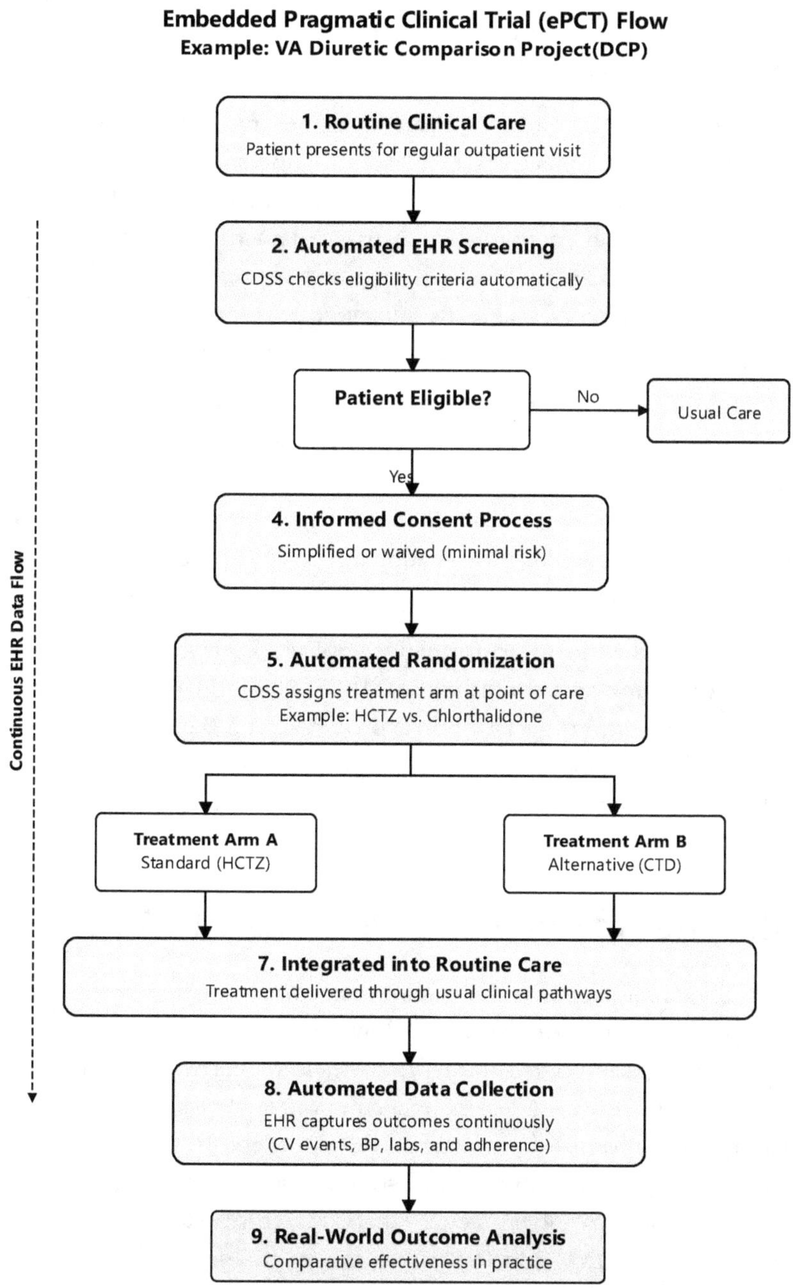


**Figure 16.1 Conceptual diagram of an embedded pragmatic clinical trial (ePCT)**

It now sustains ongoing surveillance: for instance, it automatically updates comparative effectiveness estimates for products, feeding results into NHS England's formulary review process.

In the United States, the FDA's Sentinel Initiative has evolved into a Sentinel Operations Center capable of launching prospective cohort studies within days [18]. A 2024 pilot demonstrated a 72-hour turnaround from query definition to distributed analysis across 10 data partners (covering >200 million lives) to assess myocarditis risk following a newly authorized RSV vaccine. Results were posted publicly before journal peer review, embodying "pre-publication transparency" [19].

Globally, the OHDSI network provides a technical backbone through its Common Data Model (CDM) and open-source analytics library [20]. Over 30 countries - including Japan's Medical Data Vision, South Korea's NHIS, and Brazil's SUS Analytic Platform - have adopted the OMOP CDM, enabling cross-national replication and meta-analytic pooling without data sharing.

One of the most transformative applications is **adaptive post-authorization safety studies (aPASS)**. Traditionally static, PASS are now evolving into trigger-response protocols: if a Bayesian safety signal exceeds a pre-specified threshold across ≥2 data sources, an automatic deep-dive cohort analysis is launched, reducing the reaction time from weeks to hours.

## 16.4. The Science and Practice of RWE

The credibility of real-world evidence does not flow from data volume or algorithmic sophistication alone - it emerges from the disciplined integration of scientific principles into everyday practice. This integration spans protocol design, data curation, analytical execution, regulatory interaction, and professional development. In short, RWE is both a science (grounded in causal reasoning, statistical theory, and epidemiologic design) and a practice (shaped by informatics infrastructure, workflow constraints, ethical governance, regulatory landscape, and evolving competency standards). Four interrelated dimensions are driving this convergence: (1) the deepening collaboration among historically distinct disciplines; (2) the emergence of hybrid methodological paradigms such as causal data science; (3) the layered evolution of analytical tooling; and (4) the formalization of interdisciplinary standards of practice.

### 16.4.1. Convergent Specialization in Action

RWE practice is increasingly conducted at the nexus of epidemiology, medical informatics, biostatistics, and data science - each contributing irreplaceable expertise. Rather than merging into a single discipline, these fields engage in convergent specialization: professionals develop sufficient fluency in adjacent domains to co-design and co-implement studies, while retaining core methodological rigor.

A vivid illustration is the OHDSI (Observational Health Data Sciences and Informatics) network, where a single study protocol - e.g., evaluating the comparative safety of two anticoagulants - requires:

- An **epidemiologist** to define the target trial emulation, specify time-at-risk windows, and articulate assumptions (e.g., no unmeasured confounding);
- A **medical informatician** to map phenotype algorithms to the OMOP Common Data Model across dozens of disparate databases, assess data quality flags (e.g., implausible lab values), and ensure semantic consistency (e.g., using SNOMED CT for bleeding events);
- A **biostatistician** to select appropriate estimators (e.g., high-dimensional propensity score weighting), conduct negative control analyses, and quantify uncertainty.
- A **data scientist** to orchestrate distributed execution across cloud environments, automate diagnostics, and visualize results for stakeholder review.

This model is now institutionalized: the **European Health Data Space (EHDS)** mandates that all data access requests undergo multidisciplinary review, explicitly requiring representation from epidemiology, informatics, statistics, and ethics [21].

Convergent specialization has practical consequences for how RWE is generated:

- **Protocol feasibility** is assessed before finalization - not just statistically (e.g., power), but informatically (e.g., "Is 'incident heart failure with preserved ejection fraction' reliably coded in >80 % of contributing databases?");
- **Data quality** assurance is integrated into analysis pipelines using informatics-derived metrics (e.g., temporal completeness of medication records, provider specialty consistency);
- **Regulatory submissions** increasingly include data provenance documentation (e.g., ETL logs, CDM versioning, ontology releases) alongside traditional statistical outputs.

Historically, professionals engaged in real-world evidence and data have been trained in established disciplines such as epidemiology, biostatistics, health economics, and public health. Consequently, their scholarly work has largely been disseminated through the journals and conferences of those parent fields. In less than two decades, the rapid methodological advances, regulatory integration, and expanding applications of RWE and RWD have propelled the discipline to a new threshold of maturity.

The growing technical complexity, distinct scientific identity, and specialized skill sets now demand dedicated academic and professional infrastructure - including endowed faculty positions, dedicated textbooks, discipline-specific conferences, and peer-reviewed journals. It is precisely this maturation, and the pressing need for a unified scholarly platform, that motivated the author to write this book and to establish the forthcoming *Annals of Real-World Data and Evidence (arwde.org)*. Together, these initiatives are designed to formalize the field's core principles, advance methodological standards, and provide a dedicated forum for the growing global community of RWE and RWD practitioners and researchers.

## 16.4.2. Causal Data Science: Bridging Theory and Implementation

The most significant methodological innovation of the past decade is not a new algorithm, but a new epistemology: causal data science - the disciplined application of causal inference principles within scalable computational frameworks. This paradigm recognizes that machine learning excels at prediction, but evidence generation demands identification and estimation under explicit assumptions.

Methods such as targeted maximum likelihood estimation (TMLE), double/debiased machine learning, and Bayesian causal forests operationalize this synthesis. By decoupling the flexible, high-dimensional estimation of nuisance parameters (e.g., propensity scores, outcome regressions) from the targeted, asymptotically regular estimation of causal effects, these approaches reconcile predictive machine learning with the identification rigor required for pharmacoepidemiologic inference. They enable:

- **Flexible modeling of high-dimensional confounders** (e.g., EHR-derived comorbidity trajectories, medication sequences, and healthcare utilization patterns) while preserving valid, double-robust inference;
- **Quantification of heterogeneous treatment effects** with formal uncertainty bounds, supporting precision pharmacotherapy and subgroup safety/effectiveness profiling; and
- **Computationally tractable sensitivity analyses** (e.g., E-value extensions, bias-function calibration, and partial identification bounds) that scale across millions of real-world records without compromising interpretability or regulatory-grade evidence standards.

. Regulators have increasingly articulated expectations for the rigorous use of machine learning in evidence generation. FDA's Framework for Real-World Evidence established foundational principles for evaluating real-world data fit-for-purpose, and subsequent draft guidance on artificial intelligence in drug development. It recommends that sponsors assess model credibility through risk-based evaluation of data representativeness, performance metrics with uncertainty quantification, and mitigation of algorithmic bias [22,23].

While calibration, transportability, and confounding assessment are recognized methodological considerations, they are not currently codified as universal mandatory validation criteria for regulatory submission of ML-based analyses. These evolving expectations reflect a shared regulatory priority: ensuring that computational innovation strengthens, rather than substitutes for, transparent and defensible causal inference.

## 16.4.3. Tooling Evolution: A Layered, Context-Driven Transition

The migration from SAS to R to Python is unfolding not as a clean replacement but as a layered ecosystem, where each tool serves distinct practice needs.

**Table 16.2 SAS, R and Python Ecosystem in RWE**

| Practice Layer | Dominant Tool(s) | Rationale | Current Barriers |
|---|---|---|---|
| **Regulatory Submission** | SAS (for CDISC ADaM/SDTM) | Legacy validation packs, audit trails, FDA/EMA acceptance | High cost of re-validation; lack of standardized Python submission templates |
| **Statistical Reporting & Causal Inference** | R (≈60 %), Stata (niche) | Rich ecosystem (MatchIt, survival, lme4, causalml), reproducible R Markdown workflows | Fragmentation in style guides; limited integration with cloud CI/CD |
| **Data Engineering & ML Ops** | Python (≈70 %), SQL | Scalability (Dask, Spark), FHIR/OMOP SDKs, MLflow/DVC for model governance | Need for rigorous statistical auditing of Python pipelines; less regulatory precedent |

In practice, most leading RWE units now operate hybrid pipelines. For example, the UK's OpenSAFELY platform extracts and preprocesses data in Python, performs causal analyses in R (using TargetedLearning and survey for complex survey weights), and exports final tables in SAS transport format for MHRA submissions [24]. This layered approach acknowledges that regulatory trust evolves more slowly than technical capability - and that practice must accommodate both.

Table 16.2 provides a comparison of the three ecosystems.

### 16.4.4. Formalizing Standards of Practice

As RWE matures, the field is codifying expectations for *how* evidence should be generated - not just *what* should be reported. Three initiatives illustrate this trend:

- **Competency Frameworks**: There is more support for developing a competency framework among the members of the most important professional societies and academics. The are five domains of focus: scientific rigor, data governance, technical implementation, regulatory engagement, and ethical partnership.
- **Reproducibility Standards**: The REPEAT (Reproducible Evidence: Practices to Enhance and Achieve Transparency) initiative advances RECORD by promoting transparent reporting, code sharing, and containerized workflows to support reproducible, regulator-ready real-world evidence [25].
- **Integrated Training Models**: Academic programs increasingly embed causal RWE practice. Harvard's health data science and epidemiology capstones require students to co-design protocols with clinical or regulatory partners, apply modern causal estimators to harmonized real-world datasets, and structure outputs for stakeholder review. Comparable applied tracks at Karolinska Institutet, Kyoto University, and the University of Cape Town reflect global convergence toward competency-based, computationally rigorous pharmacoepidemiology training.

**.Table 16.3 Evolving Practice Profile of an RWE Specialist**

| Practice Dimension | 2020 Typical Expectation | 2025 Emerging | 2030 Projection |
|---|---|---|---|
| **Study Design** | Define cohort/case–control using standard criteria | Specify target trial emulation with explicit transportability assumptions | Design adaptive, learning protocols with embedded randomization triggers |
| **Data Stewardship** | Extract variables via SQL; basic missingness checks | Conduct FHIR-based phenotyping; document CDM version & mapping logic; run data quality dashboards | Operate privacy-preserving federated analyses (e.g., GAIA-X, TRUSTED) with real-time provenance tracking |
| **Analytical Execution** | Fit Cox models in SAS/R; report HRs and 95 % CIs | Apply causal ML (e.g., TMLE, BART); perform E-value sensitivity; stratify by equity dimensions | Integrate ML surrogates with Bayesian calibration; auto-generate regulatory submission packages |
| **Regulatory Interaction** | Submit summary tables and narrative | Include code, data dictionaries, and negative control results in dossiers | Co-develop adaptive PASS protocols with pre-specified trigger–response rules and dashboards |
| **Professional Accountability** | IRB approval and GCP training | Document stakeholder engagement (e.g., patient advisory input); report disparity metrics | Hold certification in a competency framework; participate in cross-institutional audit networks |

Collectively, these developments signal a maturing professional identity: the RWE practitioner is no longer a statistician who occasionally uses claims data, nor a data engineer who runs scripts on EHR dumps. They are an evidence integrator - equally at ease discussing counterfactuals, FHIR resources, calibration curves, and equity impact assessments. Table 16.3 shows this evolving practice profile and future projections.

## 16.5. Converging Trends and Key Enablers

The three futures - AI-augmented analytics, real-world trials, and continuous ecosystems - are not mutually exclusive.

Their synergies are already visible: AI enhances real-world trials through improved phenotyping and dynamic sample size re-estimation; real-world trials feed high-quality, prospectively collected data into continuous ecosystems, reducing bias compared to purely observational streams; and continuous ecosystems provide the infrastructure for rapid external validation of AI models, closing the reproducibility gap.

**Table 16.4 Enablers Determining the Pace and Equity of RWE Adoption**

| Enabler | Description | Current Gaps |
|---|---|---|
| **Data governance frameworks** | Federated trust models (e.g., GAIA-X in Europe, Trusted Research Environments in the UK) that balance access with privacy. | Fragmentation across jurisdictions; limited patient representation in governance. |
| **Standards harmonization** | Global adoption of FHIR, OMOP CDM, and BRIDG for protocol representation. | Legacy claims formats (e.g., US X12) impede real-time analysis. |
| **Workforce development** | Training clinicians in RWE interpretation and data scientists in causal inference and regulatory science. | Few interdisciplinary curricula; credentialing not standardized. |
| **Incentive alignment** | Reimbursement for evidence generation (e.g., CMS's "Coverage with Evidence Development") and recognition in promotion criteria. | Short-term budgeting cycles disincentivize infrastructure investment. |
| **Patient agency** | Tools for dynamic consent, data donation, and participatory priority setting (e.g., PCORnet's Patient Engagement Studio). | Digital literacy disparities risk excluding vulnerable populations. |

Five cross-cutting enablers will determine the pace and equity of adoption. Table 16.4 summarizes these enablers.

Finally, none of these technological or methodological advances will scale without human infrastructure. The success of AI-augmented analytics, real-world trials, and continuous ecosystems depends on a maturing science-practice continuum: where causal theory informs pipeline design, and operational constraints shape methodological choices.

## 16.6. Conclusion

The future of real-world evidence is no longer a distant aspiration; it is already unfolding across clinical, regulatory, and public health arenas worldwide. Artificial intelligence is evolving beyond mere automation toward sophisticated hypothesis generation, causal inference, and even AI agents acting as (performant as) humans. Real-world trials are redefining the boundaries of feasibility, compressing timelines and expanding scale. Meanwhile, continuous evidence ecosystems are weaving RWE directly into the operational fabric of health systems, propelling us toward a genuinely learning healthcare enterprise.

Yet technological momentum alone will not carry us forward. Realizing this vision demands deliberate stewardship of fairness, transparency, and long-term sustainability. As RWE becomes increasingly ubiquitous, its enduring credibility will rest on the disciplined application of rigorous methodological standards, open cross-border collaboration, and - above all - the meaningful integration of patients as co-creators of evidence, not merely subjects of study.

Beyond these structural and ethical imperatives, the trajectory of RWE reveals a quieter, more profound phenomenon - one best understood through the physics of gravitational lensing. As RWE draws regulation, knowledge, technology, and infrastructure into its gravitational center, the boundaries around it grow beautifully indistinct. The once-rigid frontier between controlled clinical trials and real-world studies bends into a seamless continuum. The once impermeable barriers that historically isolated our data sources grow porous, softened by interoperable frameworks and privacy-preserving tokenization. And the traditionally siloed disciplines of epidemiology, pharmacoepidemiology, biostatistics, and data science increasingly intertwine, their methods and perspectives blending in practice while each retains its distinct identity.

This is not a causal displacement, but a natural property of convergence. To witness this gentle distortion of intellectual space is among the rarest privileges of our young profession - and we are fortunate not only to observe it, but to live it, shape it, and learn from it.

Moreover, the next era of RWE will not be written solely by data scientists, methodologists, or regulators. It will be co-authored by clinicians translating evidence at the bedside, by patients generating data in their homes and daily lives, and by communities advocating for health equity and representation. As our analytical capabilities expand, our moral responsibility deepens: to ensure that real-world evidence serves not only scientific advancement, but human wellbeing.

The chapters of this book have sought to equip readers with foundational knowledge, methodological tools, and practical examples. As the field accelerates, this knowledge must be continually updated, critically appraised, and ethically applied. The next chapter of RWE will be written not only by data scientists and regulators, but by clinicians at the bedside, patients in their homes, and communities advocating for health equity. The principles outlined throughout this volume - validity, relevance, transparency - remain the compass for navigating that future.

## References

1. Curtis JR, Zhang J, Saffibi S, et al. From real-world electronic health record data to real-world results using artificial intelligence. Ann Rheum Dis. 2023 Mar;82(3):306-311. doi: 10.1136/ard-2022-222834..

2. Singhal K, Azizi S, Tu T, et al. Large language models encode clinical knowledge. Nature. 2023;620(7972):169–177.

3. Regulation (EU) 2025/327 of the European Parliament and of the Council of 11 February 2025 on the European Health Data Space. Official Journal of the European Union. 2025 Feb 11;L2025/327.

4. Mariam A, Javidi H, Zabor EC, et al. Unsupervised clustering of longitudinal clinical measurements in electronic health records. PLOS Digit Health. 2024 Oct 15;3(10):e0000628.

5. Mori Y, Komura T, Adomi M, et al. Heterogeneous cardiovascular effects of sodium-glucose cotransporter 2 inhibitors in type 2 diabetes: a causal forest and target trial emulation study. Eur J Prev Cardiol. 2026 Jan 6;33(1):80-88.

6. Komorowski M, Celi LA, Badawi O, et al. The AI Clinician learns optimal treatment strategies for sepsis in intensive care. Nat Med. 2018;24(11):1716-1720.

7. Poirier C, Hswen Y, Bouzillé G, et al. Influenza forecasting for French regions combining EHR, web and climatic data sources with a machine learning ensemble approach. PLoS One. 2021 May 19;16(5):e0250890.

8. Rad MS, Huang JV, Hosseini MM, Choudhary R, Siezen H, Akabari R, et al. Deep learning for digital pathology: A critical overview of methodological framework. J Pathol Inform. 2025;19:100514.

9. U.S. Food and Drug Administration. Artificial intelligence/machine learning (AI/ML)-based software as a medical device (SaMD) action plan. Silver Spring (MD): FDA; 2021 Jan

10. Raine J, Arlett P, Cohet C, et al. The use of federated health data for signal detection: results from a HealthData@EU pilot project use case on drug-induced liver injury. Eur J Public Health. 2025 Sep 10;35(Suppl 3):iii13-iii21.

11. Collins GS, Moons KGM, Dhiman P, et al. TRIPOD+AI statement: updated guidance for reporting clinical prediction models that use regression or machine learning methods. *Lancet Digit Health.* 2024 May;6(5):e312-e325.

12. Lekadir K, Frangi AF, Porras AR, et al. FUTURE-AI: international consensus guideline for trustworthy and deployable artificial intelligence in healthcare. BMJ. 2025 Feb 5;388:e081554.

13. Jones WS, Mulder H, Wruck LM, et al. Comparative effectiveness of aspirin dosing in cardiovascular disease: the ADAPTABLE randomized clinical trial. JAMA. 2023;329(22):1968–1978.

14. Spiertz C, Lombardo G, et al. Electronic health records (EHRs) in clinical research and platform trials: Application of the innovative EHR-based methods developed by EU-PEARL. J Biomed Inform. 2024 Jan;149:104567.

15. Vogel C, Handels RLH, et al. ROADMAP: Real-world Outcomes across the Alzheimer's Disease spectrum for better care: Multi-modal data Access Platforms. J Prev Alzheimers Dis. 2020;7(4):224-232.

16. Ishani A, Leatherman SM, Woods P, et al. Design of a pragmatic clinical trial embedded in the Electronic Health Record: The VA's Diuretic Comparison Project. Contemp Clin Trials. 2022;116:106754.

17. Williamson EJ, Walker AJ, Bhaskaran K, et al. OpenSAFELY: factors associated with COVID-19 death in 17 million patients. Nature. 2020;584(7821):430–436.

18. Platt R, Carnahan R, Brown JS, et al. The evolving Sentinel System: from passive monitoring to active trial infrastructure. Clin Pharmacol Ther. 2024;115(2):302–310.

19. U.S. Food and Drug Administration. FDA announces major steps to implement real-time clinical trials. Silver Spring (MD): FDA; 2026 Apr 28.

20. Hripcsak G, Duke JD, Shah NH, et al. Observational Health Data Sciences and Informatics (OHDSI): opportunities for observational researchers. Stud Health Technol Inform. 2015;216:574–578.

21. Regulation (EU) 2025/327 of the European Parliament and of the Council of 11 February 2025 on the European Health Data Space and amending Directive 2011/24/EU and Regulation (EU) 2024/2847. Official Journal of the European Union, L 2025/327.

22. U.S. Food and Drug Administration. Considerations for the Use of Artificial Intelligence To Support Regulatory Decision-Making for

Drug and Biological Product Submissions: Draft Guidance for Industry and FDA Staff. Silver Spring, MD: FDA; 2025 Jan.

23. European Medicines Agency. Reflection paper on the use of Artificial Intelligence (AI) in the medicinal product lifecycle. EMA/CHMP/CVMP/83833/2023. London: EMA; 2024 Sep.

24. Curtis HJ, Croker R, Walker AJ, et al. OpenSAFELY: a platform for analysing electronic health records designed for reproducible research. Pharmacoepidemiol Drug Saf. 2024;33(2):e5815. doi:10.1002/pds.5815.

25. Wang SV, Sreedhara SK, Schneeweiss S, et al. Reproducibility of real-world evidence studies using clinical practice data to inform regulatory and coverage decisions. Nat Commun. 2022;13:5126.

# Afterword

The chapters that precede this page have sought to equip you with foundational knowledge, methodological rigor, and practical frameworks for navigating the complexities of real-world evidence. Yet as the field accelerates, static knowledge is insufficient. The science of RWE demands continuous updating, critical appraisal, and unwavering ethical application. What is cutting-edge today becomes baseline tomorrow; what is uncertain today will be resolved through the very practices outlined here.

Through every shift in technology, every expansion of data scale, and every convergence of disciplines, the principles detailed throughout this volume remain your compass. Validity ensures that our inferences withstand scrutiny. Relevance guarantees that our questions matter to those they affect. Transparency sustains trust across borders, institutions, and belief systems. Hold these close as you move forward.

This volume was conceived not as a solitary work, but as the first pillar of a cohesive scholarly arc. Real-world evidence has matured into a discipline that deserves its own dedicated literature - distinct from, yet informed by, epidemiology, biostatistics, health economics, and data science. To that end, companion volumes are in development to deepen specific domains of practice:

*Real-World Data: Sources and Standards* will provide a systematic taxonomy of data provenance, fitness assessment, linkage strategies, as well as data networks and analytical platforms across traditional and emerging sources. *Real-World Evidence: Tools and Templates* will offer reproducible frameworks for study design, protocol development, analysis planning, data collection, data analysis, and reporting - designed for immediate application. *Real-World Evidence: Methods and Mastery* will advance the methodological frontier, addressing causal inference, bias mitigation, and hybrid and adaptive designs in complex evidence ecosystems. Finally, *Real-World Medicine: Diseases & Drugs* will translate clinical and therapeutic concepts into precise, accessible language for RWE practitioners who must engage with medical content beyond their immediate specialty.

These works are not sequels in a commercial sense, but methodological companions - each addressing a distinct layer of the evidence generation lifecycle. Together, they aim to provide the integrated literacy that our discipline now requires.

This book is also accompanied by a structured scholarly ecosystem at evidencemastery.com: curated guidelines, interactive data source explorations, and AI-assisted utilities designed to support rigorous workflow. Periodic masterclasses and, in time, the *Annals of Real-World Data and Evidence* - a peer-reviewed journal dedicated to methodological innovation and ethical stewardship - will extend this commitment to collective advancement with the emphasis of being industry inclusive and not just academic. These resources exist to organize a field that has expanded faster than its training infrastructure, and to equip practitioners with reproducible, decision-ready frameworks.

They are offered not as endpoints, but as invitations: to deepen your practice, to connect with a global community of peers, and to contribute your voice to the evolving story of real-world evidence. If any part of this journey resonates, you are welcome to explore these resources at evidencemastery.com. Access is open; what is required is only curiosity and a commitment to advancing evidence that matters.

The work of generating real-world evidence is inherently collective, iterative, and forward-looking. I hope this volume serves not as a conclusion, but as a foundation - a shared starting point for the conversations, studies, and innovations yet to come. Thank you for walking this path with me. I look forward to continuing it, together.

Massoud Toussi

# Index

## D



## E

## I



## J



## L



## M



## N



## O

## P



## Q



## R

## S



## T



## V



## W

# About the author

**Massoud Toussi, MD, PhD, MBA**, is a globally recognized leader at the intersection of real-world evidence, pharmacoepidemiology, and healthcare innovation. For more than two decades, he has shaped the scientific, operational, and strategic foundations of RWE across pharmaceutical companies, contract research organizations, regulatory frameworks, and academic collaborations worldwide.

Currently Vice President of Real-World Evidence at United Biosource Corporation (UBC), Dr. Toussi has designed, led, or overseen hundreds of studies spanning every major therapeutic area. His work is distinguished not only by scale, but by a steadfast commitment to methodological rigor and translational relevance. He is a co-author of seminal resources that have helped define global standards in the field, including the *ENCePP Methodological Guide*, the *HARmonized Protocol Template (HARPER)*, and *The PASS Book*.

Beyond study execution, Dr. Toussi advises multinational organizations on evidence strategy, scientific communication, and sustainable business development - always with an eye toward advancing patient-centered outcomes and health system learning. He is also the founder of the **Evidence Mastery™** learning ecosystem, a curated platform of tools, masterclasses, and community resources dedicated to empowering the next generation of evidence leaders.

*Real-World Evidence: Principles and Practice* embodies his enduring mission: to elevate global understanding of RWE and RWD, to demystify complexity without compromising precision, and to equip professionals at every stage of their journey with the clarity, confidence, and ethical grounding needed to generate evidence that truly matters.

www.ingramcontent.com/pod-product-compliance
Lightning Source LLC
LaVergne TN
LVHW052037200926
848481LV00005B/1709